Natural Remedies in

Parkinson's Disease

Dr. Rafael Gonzalez Maldonado

Natural Remedies in

Parkinson's Disease

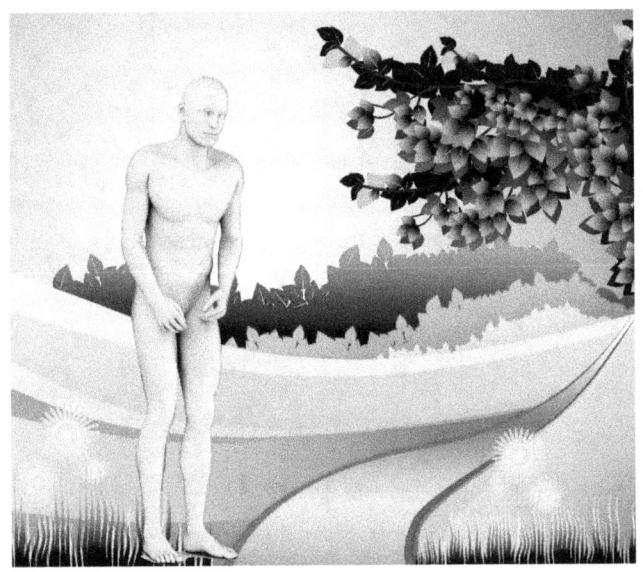

Dr. Rafael Gonzalez Maldonado

TITLE: *Natural Remedies in Parkinson's Disease*

AUTHOR: *Rafael Gonzalez Maldonado*

Edited: Createspace (Amazon), North Charleston

1st. Edition: February 2017.

Translated by Claire Huttlinger

ISBN 13: 978-1543090000

ISBN 10: 1543090001

WARNING: DISCLAIMER. *The below uses are based on tradition, scientific theories, or limited research. They often have not been thoroughly tested in humans, and safety and effectiveness have not always been proven. Some of these conditions are potentially serious, and should be evaluated by a qualified healthcare provider. There may be other proposed uses that are not listed below. The concepts and data in this book are not optional suggestions or recommendations but subject to errors or guesses debatable, and must be contrasted with the judgment of the physician. This information is not specific medical advice and just try to help clarify health concerns; are based on review of scientific research data, historical practice patterns, and clinical experience should not be followed by a patient or acquaintance without consulting the responsible physician must consider each individual case, with the history, medications and patient's clinical situation and monitor inconsistencies or errors in dose*

To Rosa

...and I drank strong wine,
the way the champions of pleasure drink.

(C.P. Cavafi: "I went", 1913)

Index

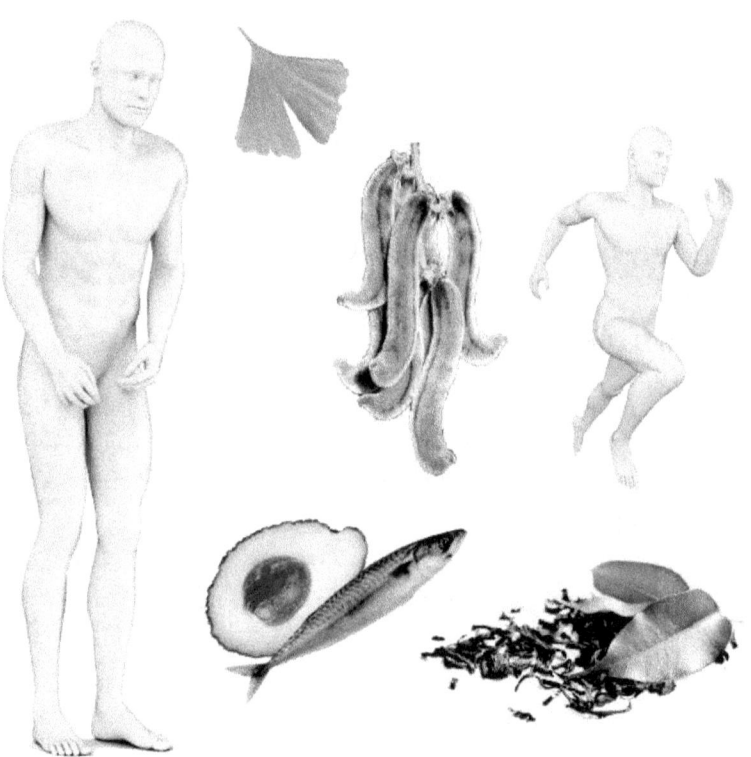

Introduction

Natural levodopa from mucuna has advantages over Sinemet. Anti-parkinson's treatment often causes daytime sleepiness that is relieved with ginkgo. Passiflora calms patients without the problems caused by benzodiazepines. Bacopa improves memory. Ginseng prevents drops in blood pressure. Green tea increases the effect of medications. Plantago supports regularity. Healing benefits are obtained from diets, massages and music. Outdoor exercise is the best prevention ...

Half of people with Parkinson's disease use natural remedies[153]. They are sold in herbalists' shops or online and many are dispensed in such low concentrations that they only serve as placebos. Others are effective and may even be dangerous in sensitive patients or when combined with pharmaceuticals.

Doctors, aware of the reality that patients are turning to self-treatment through home remedies, have a range of reactions. Some physicians prefer to ignore the problem: they don't ask, and the patient does not tell. Others speak with contempt about complementary therapies having no documentation to support them (in the words of Spanish philosopher Antonio Machado, "*People scorn what they know nothing about*"), and the patient continues to self-medicate in secret. The third possibility is to speak openly with patients, allowing them to express their thoughts about the natural therapies that they choose, to understand how desperately they seek some kind of relief, and to offer guidance about what is contraindicated or, in our opinion, useless, and what could produce benefits.

Doctors should be familiar with natural remedies and communicate to their patients that they are not a replacement for medication. They are not alternative but rather complementary treatment therapies. Patients will comply if they see that their doctors are advising them from an informed standpoint. Parkinson's patients are especially attuned to whether or not their physicians are informed, and to how much they know about a remedy being recommended or discouraged.

Complementary therapies are proposed for Parkinson's disease based on their antioxidant or neuroprotective properties or for their ability to increase dopamine and other neurotransmitters. We must add, however, that many other remedies relieve the uncomfortable symptoms of Parkinson's.

What we need is to alleviate the symptoms. For example, tremor decreases if anxiety is relieved by a natural sedative. The constipation commonly associated with Parkinson's is counteracted physiologically by certain plants that increase bowel movement, and this will result in an increased absorption of drugs. Tisanes that facilitate sleep are preferred over benzodiazepines. Some natural infusions prevent drops in blood pressure that are characteristic of the disease, and often drug-induced. Other natural substances increase alertness, improve attention and avoid daytime sleepiness.

Patients who use complementary therapies tend to be more attentive to their treatment routines (including conventional drugs and rehabilitation) and take a more active role in confronting the disease.

Because human clinical trials of complementary therapies are limited by the variability of products, concentrations and doses, far more studies use laboratory animals. For these, researchers use experimental models involving toxins that damage the nervous system and produce symptoms that mimic those seen in Parkinson's disease.

There are natural remedies that may have only modest benefits in patients but open up new therapeutic pathways, for example, turmeric, baroca or cannabis: by studying their modes of action related molecules can be investigated, giving rise to new drugs for the treatment of Parkinson's disease.

Finally, I wish to reiterate that a product, simply by virtue of being natural, is not necessarily safe or effective. Even when it *is* effective (i.e., it produces effects) it can have unwanted side effects in addition to the desired primary benefits. What we buy could work only as a placebo, be totally ineffective, or simply be a scam.

No natural remedy should be purchased if not clearly labeled by the manufacturer regarding its contents, ingredients and concentrations, the recommended doses, and all possible incompatibilities or interactions.

Complementary therapies are big business and many products are sold without sufficient controls; often they do not clarify the composition or simply do not contain what they claim to. Patients should always consult an informed medical professional before using natural remedies.

Rafael González Maldonado.

Granada, February 2017.

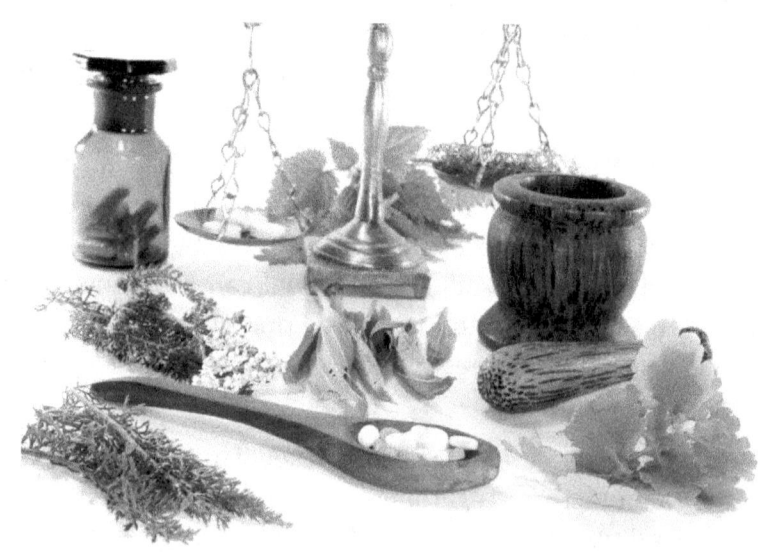

Alternative versus complementary medicine

Unlike "alternative" treatments, complementary medicine does not attempt to replace conventional medicine, but should be used to supplement it with natural remedies.

I. Basic Concepts

Natural remedies have been used since antiquity and initially were prescribed by conventional physicians of the day. Later, with the development of scientific medicine, these natural products were passed over in favor of pharmaceuticals, although many of these had their origins in plants or natural substances.

Beginning in the 1970s, a swell of popular opinion supported the rejection of conventional treatments in favor of a return to natural principles. The concept of alternative medicine developed as a separate option. Fortunately, in recent times, this movement has evolved into a philosophy that views complementary and integrative medicine as a supplement to conventional therapy.

ALTERNATIVE MEDICINE

Alternative medicine is any practice that claims to have the healing effects of medicine but is not supported by evidence obtained through the scientific method, such that a product's effectiveness has not been proven beyond the placebo effect.[160] It consists of a wide range of practices, products and "therapies" including new or traditional pseudo-medical procedures.

COMPLEMENTARY AND INTEGRATIVE MEDICINE

Complementary medicine is alternative medicine that is used along with evidence-based medicine in the belief, not always proven by scientific methods, that it enhances the treatment. Integrative medicine is the combination of practices and methods of alternative and complementary medicine with scientific medicine.[400, 630]

NATUROPATHY

Naturopathy is best described as a philosophy of life and uses other techniques or healing methods provided they are based in natural elements. Health is found in nature. Healthy living involves eating natural foods and drinking pure water, getting daily exercise, avoiding excesses, and learn to relax.

All doctors, from Hippocrates to the most fanatical defenders of conventional medicine, agree with recommendations such as these. The only difference is that naturopaths give much more importance to these natural remedies and prefer to avoid pharmaceutical drugs.

Naturopathy is as old as medicine, but began to be developed independently in the nineteenth century, when advances in surgery and new drugs made many people forget the benefits of natural remedies.

NATUROPATHY IN TREATING PARKINSON'S DISEASE

We have said that Naturopathy is a philosophy of life. In a naturopathic perspective of Parkinson's disease, patients have to assimilate these general principles, which should be integrated gradually into their personal lifestyles. Natural remedies described in this book will be an important part of treatment, without giving up conventional drugs, although these could be reduced at times.

Some advocate that diseases correspond to basic models of psychic performance.[209] Parkinson's disease is associated with a strong desire to dominate and control everything and everyone, instead of living in an atmosphere of love, tolerance and understanding. It is considered that Parkinson's patients have thought processes that are rigid and limited, lacking in creativity, and slow to change; these characteristics are in accordance with paralyzing and stagnant models of reasoning.

To apply a more positive view, the disease itself may represent an opportunity for growth, giving way to a more meaningful life. A person's mental attitude and emotional-psychological integration with the body as a whole is essential.

NATURAL PRODUCTS AND REMEDIES

Most complementary therapies are based on natural products or remedies in which herbs (phytotherapy), nutrients (including vitamins) and special diets are included. Other unconventional therapies such as massage, aromatherapy, music, and techniques of self-discipline are also considered.

That is the orientation of our book: to consider the possibility that those complementary, as opposed to alternative, therapies based on natural (non-pharmacological) remedies, may contribute to the treatment of Parkinson's disease.

We accomplish this with two essential considerations: first, the use of natural remedies must be integrated with drug treatment, and second, it must always be supervised by the patient's physician who will assess the effectiveness of the remedies and monitor for any contraindications or interactions.

SCIENTIFIC EVIDENCE

Many natural remedies are increasingly undergoing scientifically proven clinical research.

The difficulties are many: the lack of confidence on the part of a large portion of the medical community, and the diversity of presentations and concentrations of the natural products under investigation, are just two of the obstacles. Nevertheless, we are seeing a growing body of protocol-based research involving controlled, randomized, and double-blind studies supporting many of the remedies detailed here.

Although publication of research in humans is relatively rare, there is extensive work in cell culture studies and laboratory animals (mainly rats, mice, nematodes and flies).

These natural remedies are tested on animals that have undergone procedures reproducing the mechanisms of the disease, known as "animal models of Parkinson's disease". Protocols are also developed to determine the effects they produce.

ANIMAL MODELS FOR RESEARCH

Human clinical trials and studies in laboratory animals (*in vivo*) and cell cultures (*in vitro*) are performed to investigate the effects of natural remedies.

In animals, various "models" that mimic the pathology to be investigated are used. In Parkinson's disease dopaminergic neurons are affected, typically those of the substantia nigra and the striatum. Studies use mice (or other animals) and administer a toxin (MPTP, 6-OHDA, rotenone or Paraquat) that causes lesions in the targeted brain nuclei inducing a state of parkinsonism.[54, 318]

There are other animal models in which parkinsonism is produced through genetic modifications. The best known is the case of the fruit fly (*Drosophila melanogaster*) that have large, easily manipulated chromosomes, a short life span (one month) and many offspring. Genes of the Drosophila are altered to cause deposits of alpha-synuclein in the neurons, imitating what takes place in Parkinson's disease.[153] In other genetic manipulations mice are used.

In recent years studies on genetics and nervous system development are conducted using a nematode (a worm with no rings) called *Caenorhabditis elegans*. The worm body is cylindrical, semi-transparent and formed of simple organs and systems. The genome of the nematode is well known, and it has two forms of reproduction: hermaphroditic and hete-rosexual (the male has a copulatory tail) which favors greater genetic variability.

Whatever the method employed, when parkinsonism is induced animals lose mobility and cognitive capacities and their behavior is altered. The mechanisms by which the drugs or natural substances prevent or improve these neural injuries and symptoms are then studied.

It is relatively easy to evaluate mobility. To assess memory loss or other cognitive functions a maze or learning test is used.

It is more difficult to discern how "depressed" a mouse is. Mood is deduced by basal activity (as compared to a typical model) or quality of relationship, and measured by the responsiveness to stress tests. All these methods are systematized and experimentally sound.

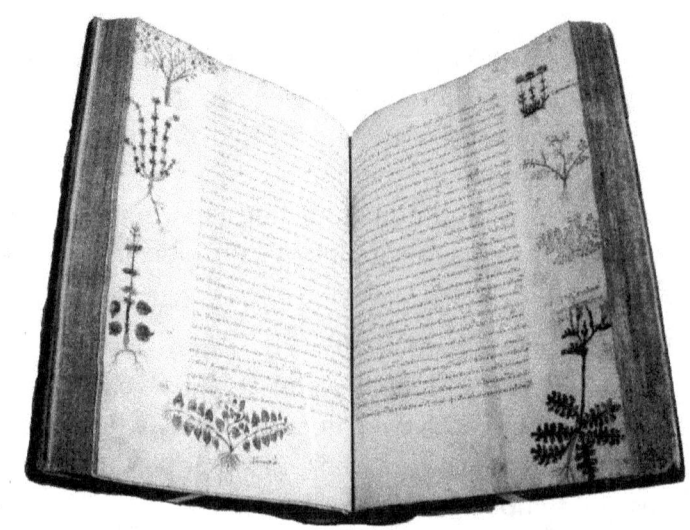

Dioscorides: *De Materia Medica.*

Codex manuscript, XV century, Byzantium.

This book includes 600 medicinal plants.

II. Phytotherapy (herbs and plants)

Levodopa was hidden in legumes until 1913 when it was discovered by Marcus Guggenheim[190], and now it comes in blue tablets known as Sinemet. The scientist became dizzy and vomited after eating some beans he had cultivated himself, and then he wanted to analyze what those plants contained. It was another milestone for herbal medicine, phytotherapy: in Greek, *fyto* means plant and *therapeia* is translated as treatment.

Herbal medicine uses the healing properties of plants. Those who prescribe the natural forms of them are sometimes called shamans or quacks, but when a laboratory extracts the active ingredient from the same plant, and patents and markets it, this is considered a scientific breakthrough.

An herb is more than its main active ingredient. They contain numerous substances that act synergistically. The herbalist prescribes according to the patient's individual characteristics, lifestyle and the other, co-occurring symptoms. We have moved from an era of philosophical confrontation to one in which scientific medicine works with traditional remedies. Now pharmaceutical companies are investigating new preparations obtained from plants used in traditional medicine.[612]

PRECAUTIONS WITH HERBS

There are official warnings[631] about using St. John's Wort and other herbal products that are sold freely. Herbs are not harmless. They contain chemicals that can have side effects, cause interactions with other drugs, or produce undesirable clinical situations that the doctor should be aware of.[227]

One of the most frequent impacts of medicinal plants is that they can interfere with blood clotting (sometimes beneficially), either alone or in combination with other drugs. This occurs with, in a greater or lesser degree, garlic, ginger, hypericum, green tea and turmeric, among others,[357] and the physician should take into account each patient's exposure to these substances.

HERBS IN PARKINSON'S DISEASE

The ancients employed the plant thornapple or Devil's snare (*Datura stramonium*) to treat tremor thanks to its anticholinergic effect (similar to Akineton or Artane). Common beans (*Vicia Fava*) and other exotic legumes such as velvet beans (*Mucuna pruriens*) contain levodopa and for centuries they have been used to treat what is now known as Parkinson's disease.[389] Ergot (*Claviceps purpurea*) is a fungus that grows on grains from which dopamine agonists (agent that activates the body's receptors to elicit a response) such as bromocriptine (Parlodel) and pergolide (Pharken) can be obtained. Another antiparkinsonian medication, selegiline (Eldepryl) is a monoamine oxidase inhibitor, a similar substance to the one found in the leaves of tobacco (*Nicotiana tabacum*) and banisterine (*Banisteria caapi*) plants.[633]

Beans

All neurologists know that common beans (*Vicia fava*) contain levodopa. Their plantlets, pods and seeds accommodate this natural amino acid which passes into the brain where it is converted to dopamine.[213]

Common beans improve Parkinson's symptoms. When patients who experience fluctuating spikes in symptoms eat beans, their on-periods (alleviated symptoms) are prolonged[24] and this clinical improvement parallels with the rise in blood levels of levodopa.[441] Eating beans customarily can be a useful treatment for the Parkinson's patients with mild symptoms[440] provided they do not experience favism.

The concentration of levodopa in common beans is low. A patient would need such a large daily amount it would be unfeasible, not to mention the accompanying flatulence. However, bean sprouts germinated in the dark have a much higher concentration of levodopa, as well as natural carbidopa, according to a recent study.[363] When these bean sprouts are consumed, patients experience distinct improvement in motor activity, higher than expected, but an excessive dose may produce dyskinesias. It is suggested that, like mucuna, these sprouts also contain other enhancing substances. Medication should then be adjusted by a neurologist.

The second possibility is to add carbidopa (which in the U.S. is sold independently under the name Lodosyn) as was done in an earlier study.[261] Clinical responses and levodopa plasma levels in 6 patients treated with conventional levodopa/carbidopa (Sinemet) were compared after giving 100-200 g of cooked bean sprouts with an additional 25-50 mg of carbidopa. At 39 minutes (on average) they had a clinical improvement similar to those treated with Sinemet and also much more lasting: 285 minutes with beans compared to 75 minutes with the conventional medication. These researchers suggest that beans can replace other protein-rich foods to avoid motor oscillations in levodopa-treated patients.

Finally, there is a third option, a tropical bean which naturally contains high concentrations of levodopa: *Mucuna pruriens,* discussed below.

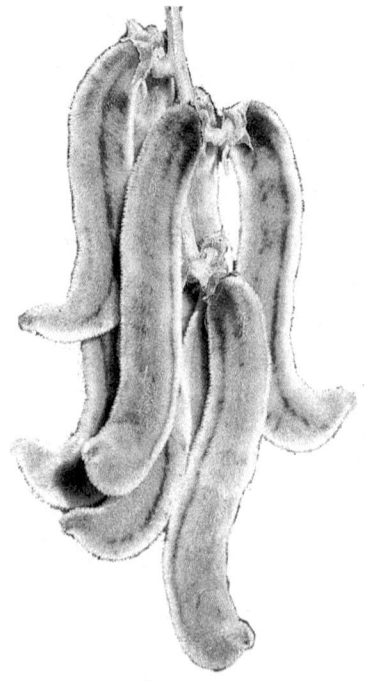

Mucuna pruriens is a tropical bean containing large amounts of natural levodopa, known by many in the field as L-DOPA. Famous neurologists have patented methods of extraction for its advantages over the synthetic forms, Sinemet and Madopar. This natural levodopa is less toxic and has a faster and more lasting effect, and can delay the need for pharma-ceuticals and combination therapies. Mucuna should always be taken under medical supervision.

Mucuna

I first tried mucuna seed powder in the Brazilian Amazon. A woman with Parkinson's disease, being treated with mucuna, had invited me to Manaus to see her. I adjusted her dose of mucuna, and added green tea to her regimen (to enhance its effect). Observing her dramatic improvement, I took the same combination and I felt euphoric and hyperactive. Mucuna indeed seemed to work, I had experienced it myself.

Mucuna pruriens is a variety of bean that grows in the tropics and, because of its high content in levodopa, is the most important natural remedy for Parkinson's disease. Mucuna deserves a separate section and will be addressed in an essay[176] further on; here we will review the most important issues.

Four thousand years before the birth of James Parkinson, patients with Parkinson's symptoms were identified in India. They were diagnosed with *Kampa-vata*, a disease characterized by tremor (*kampa* in Sanskrit) and is classified by Ayurveda among the neurological disorders (*Vata rogas*).[331, 333]

The patients were treated with levodopa which was obtained by crushing the seeds of *Mucuna pruriens*, a climbing legume in the rain forests of Asia and America. Its reddish and hairy pods cause pain and itching (*pruriens* means pruritus in Latin) to those who dare to touch them. Mucuna seeds contain a great deal of natural levodopa and probably other active components that can improve symptoms of Parkinson's disease.[190, 330, 568]

FUNDAMENTALS

Scientific journals eventually began publishing cases of patients with Parkinson's disease that improve after eating common beans or mucuna. The Parkinson's Disease Study Group undertook a multi-center clinical trial in

60 patients[419], of which 26 were taking Sinemet before the test and other 34 were "pharmacologically virgins" (they had never taken levodopa).

All of them were treated for 12 weeks with powder from mucuna seeds, an average of 6 scoops, each containing 7.5 grams, equivalent to 250 mg of levodopa. In other words, each scoop contained the same amount of levodopa as a tablet of Sinemet 250/25, but without carbidopa. Neurologists of four centers screened patients using the appropriate scales (UPDRS) and found considerable improvement that was statistically confirmed.[419] Thus, Ayurveda medicinal recipes have demonstrated their clinical effectiveness.

THE MACUNA-BASED MEDICINE ZANDOPA

This legume seems to work. Based on evidence from research, mucuna seed powder (called HP-200) was marketed as a drug under the brand name Zandopa[332]. It was first distributed in India and has been available in the United Kingdom since 2008. Now customers can buy it freely online without a prescription. It is important to be careful, however, because the dose of levodopa is relatively high (250 mg per dose) when combined with carbidopa or other antiparkinsonian treatments (see below).

DOUBLE AND TRIPLE SUCCESS WITH MICE

We can experimentally induce parkinsonism (unilateral or bilateral) in rodents via certain toxic substances. Used in these trials, levodopa from mucuna has no side effects and produces an improvement that is double or triple that of the synthetic version.[222, 330] This also suggests that mucuna can contain components that enhance the action of levodopa (as when combined with carbidopa, entacapone or tolcapone). There is another possibility: namely that mucuna itself, regardless of its levodopa content, relieves the symptoms of Parkinson's.

In another experiment, animals ate macuna extract for a year. They were then put down and their neurotransmitters were measured in different areas of their brains. Interestingly, no changes were seen in the nigrostriatal pathway, but dopamine was significantly increased in the cerebral cortex.[332]

EXTRACTS OF MUCUNA PATENTED BY NEUROLOGISTS

Ayurveda recipes have drawn the attention of several neurologists since 1990, and they launched serious clinical studies which have subsequently confirmed the benefits of Indian herbs.

Experiments with rats have also shown that natural levodopa improved symptoms and produced less neurological damage than the synthetic version. It was concluded that extracts of *Mucuna pruriens* contain high concentrations of levodopa and are more effective and better tolerated with fewer side effects.

Obviously no one can, at this point, "invent" *Mucuna pruriens* treatment as it has existed for thousands of years in India. Some, however, have patented[115, 299] certain techniques for extracting levodopa and other substances found in these legumes. These physicians provide documentation in their patents which conclude that the use of these extracts of mucuna have advantages over the conventional treatment with synthetic levodopa (Sinemet or Madopar).

APPLICATIONS OF MUCUNA

Renowned specialists who study mucuna have evidence that these extracts may be useful in the treatment of multiple neurodegenerative processes, and have applications for almost everything they treat. Specifically, researchers have recorded the potential benefits of using extracts of mucuna for chorea, Parkinson's and Alzheimer's diseases, and vascular dementia;[115] further applications include disnutrition and many other metabolic disorders and systemic endocrine and autoimmune disturbances (vitamin deficiency, lupus, demyelinating disease, etc.), as well as neurotoxic, ischemic or traumatic injuries.[299]

BENEFITS OF NATURAL OVER CONVENTIONAL LEVODOPA

Based on the references provided, fundamental information in the patent reveals that the extracts of mucuna have several important advantages over standard levodopa-carbidopa medications (Sinemet) or levodopa-benserazide (Madopar).

A WIDE THERAPEUTIC WINDOW

A therapeutic window is what we call the range of dosage in which a drug can be used without causing toxic effects, and this window is wider in mucuna. That means that there is a large variability between the minimally effective dose of mucuna and one that could cause damage in the body.

FASTER AND MORE DURABLE BENEFITS

Researchers gave patients a tablet of Sinemet and they noticed an "on" effect period (reduction in symptoms) initiated after 54 minutes. But when subjects took mucuna the effect began after only 23-27 minutes.[259]

In addition to being quick-acting, mucuna (at a dose of 30 g) has been found to be effective for longer durations: patients were still "on" for 204 minutes after taking the seed extract, surpassing the Sinemet tablet by half an hour.[259]

REDUCED TOXICITY OF NATURAL LEVODOPA

Neither acute nor chronic toxic effects have been described. Even with high doses of mucuna there were fewer adverse effects, such as nausea and abdominal discomfort, than in patients who received the equivalent of the conventional drugs.[115]

Other long-term studies of mucuna (in monkeys and rats) have shown that the dreaded dyskinesias and other symptoms associated with continuous treatment with levodopa are reduced, and in some cases even dramatically.[306, 307]

POTENTIAL DELAY OF COMBINATION THERAPY

This statement appears in the preamble of the patent application.[115] A professor of phytotherapy and two neurologists believe that mucuna alone may suffice to relieve patients' symptoms for a period of time, and therefore combination therapy (levodopa plus agonists) can be delayed.

SYNTHETIC LEVODOPA AND NATURAL LEVODOPA

Synthetic levodopa (Sinemet or Madopar) is not sold in pure form, but is combined with substances that make it more effective: inhibitors of dopa-decarboxylase (carbidopa or benserazide).

Mucuna contains natural levodopa but not (theoretically) carbidopa or benserazide. This levodopa from mucuna should be given in greater quantities, by four to five times, to obtain clinical efficacy similar to that of conventional drugs, Sinemet or Madopar. One tablet of Sinemet (250 mg levodopa and 25 mg carbidopa) or one tablet of Madopar (levodopa 200 mg and 50 mg benserazide) induce the same clinical effect as 1000 mg of natural levodopa from mucuna.

HIGH COST OF MUCUNA

Mucuna preparations usually sold online contain small amounts of levodopa. Furthermore, it is not combined with (carbidopa-like) "enhancers" and so has hardly any effect on symptoms.

As previously stated, in order to achieve the clinical effect of a tablet of Madopar or Sinemet, 1000 mg of levodopa mucuna must be given. That would be like 4 scoops (30 g of seed powder) of Zandopa or nearly 17 capsules of other preparations providing 60 mg per dose.

For example, a patient taking four daily tablets of Sinemet or Madopar who wants to switch to mucuna alone would need 4000 mg natural levodopa daily, i.e .120 mg of seed powder (a bottle of Zandopa contains 175 mg) or 66 capsules of Bonusan (60 mg levodopa each) or 40 cápsules of Solbia (100 mg levodopa each). Few patients want to take on such a cost.

The problem is further complicated by the fact that the actual content of levodopa in many products sold online is lower than stated on the label.[534]

ADDING CARBIDOPA TO MUCUNA

The synthetic levodopa in Sinemet is enhanced by carbidopa. This increases its clinical effectiveness and prevents peripheral side effects (nausea, tachycardia).

Carbidopa further improves the effects of mucuna: it reduces the mild side effects and doubles or triples its effectiveness. This factor must be taken into account when a patient combines mucuna and Sinemet (or Madopar or Stalevo): the carbidopa in these drugs also interacts with the natural levodopa in mucuna by strengthening its clinical effects, and the dose should be greatly reduced.

And what happens when the patient does not take Sinemet or other drugs? Then mucuna may be insufficient. These patients complain that mucuna "does not do anything" and this is due to the fact that their decarboxylase is quickly removed from the blood, without allowing time for a sufficient amount to reach the brain.

The solution seems to be to add carbidopa, which in some countries is sold separately (as Lodosyn). When Lodosyn is not available, there is the option of taking half a tablet of Sinemet Plus (12.5 mg carbidopa) and subtract the amount of synthetic levodopa (50 mg), taking into account that it will now be more potent.

ENHANCING LEVODOPA

One inexpensive and clinically effective option is to use levodopa enhancers that are contained in conventional drugs.

It is a good idea to mix the mucuna seed powder with very low doses of Madopar (e.g. half a tablet in the morning and half at night). Thus, only 200 mg of synthetic levodopa are provided, but this has the advantage that there are 50 mg of benserazide included. This will greatly enhance the effectiveness of natural levodopa in the added mucuna.

One can also add green tea; its polyphenols are inhibitors of decarboxylase (such as benserazide or carbidopa), further reinforcing the levodopa. The overall bioavailability of levodopa will be improved. In some patients a spectacular result has been obtained, as we have previously published.[179,180]

RISKS OF COMBINING MUCUNA AND GREEN TEA

Green tea enhances the effect of beans in general and of mucuna in particular. This effect can also be seen in patients taking Sinemet or Madopar: it is recommended that patients be aware of this phenomenon due to the increase in potency it can produce.

Carbidopa-like effect. There is something in green tea that acts like carbidopa. It contains polyphenols which inhibit dopa-decarboxylase,[47] an action similar to that carried out by the carbidopa or benserazide contained in Sinemet or Madopar.

Entacapone-like effect. In addition, there is something that acts like entacapone in green tea. Ponifenol, EGCG (Epi-Gallo-Catecin-gallate) promotes the entry into the brain of levodopa and prolongs its bioavailability in the bloodstream because it inhibits the COMT enzyme.[254]

This action is similar to that of entacapone; namely, that beans mixed with green tea have Stalevo-like effects, but with different proportions. Obviously, if you take levodopa (mucuna or otherwise), its effectiveness will be reinforced and this should be taken into account as there is risk of overdose. Always consult your doctor.

These "carbidopa-like" and "entacapone-like" effects can be seen with green tea and they are independent of their other neuroprotective benefits[191] so the tea is recommended for many Parkinson's patients.

LEVODOPA

Mucuna has such diverse and numerous healing properties that it cannot be explained by levodopa alone. Studies in patients and in laboratory animals show that *Mucuna pruriens* has other ingredients that demonstrate exceptional characteristics. Therefore, it must contain other substances that enhance absorption of levodopa and metabolic efficiency.

These substances, identified or not, confer special potency on mucuna, perhaps boosting the levodopa or adding some kind of dopamine agonist and even extended its effects. More research in this area is needed.

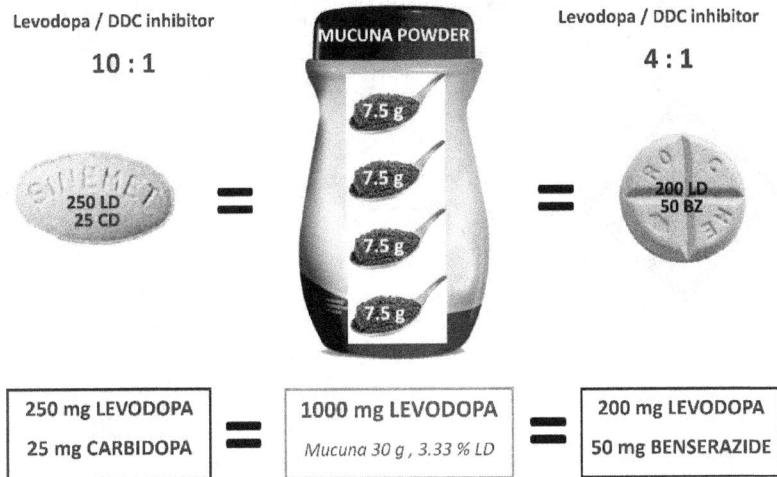

Levodopa / DDC inhibitor 10 : 1		Levodopa / DDC inhibitor 4 : 1
250 mg LEVODOPA 25 mg CARBIDOPA	1000 mg LEVODOPA *Mucuna 30 g , 3.33 % LD*	200 mg LEVODOPA 50 mg BENSERAZIDE

COMPLEXITIES OF ADJUSTING MUCUNA

As mucuna seed powder does not contain carbidopa (theoretically) the clinical effectiveness of 1000 mg of it natural levodopa is equivalent to a tablet of Sinemet 250/25 or of Madopar 200/50.

Illustration: *González-Maldonado R, González-Redondo R, Di Caudo C. The clinical effects of mucuna and green tea in combination with levodopa-benserazide in advanced Parkinson's disease: Experience from a case report. International Parkinson and Movement Disorders Society, Berlin June 2016. Mov Disord 2016; 31 Suppl 2, pp. S639..*

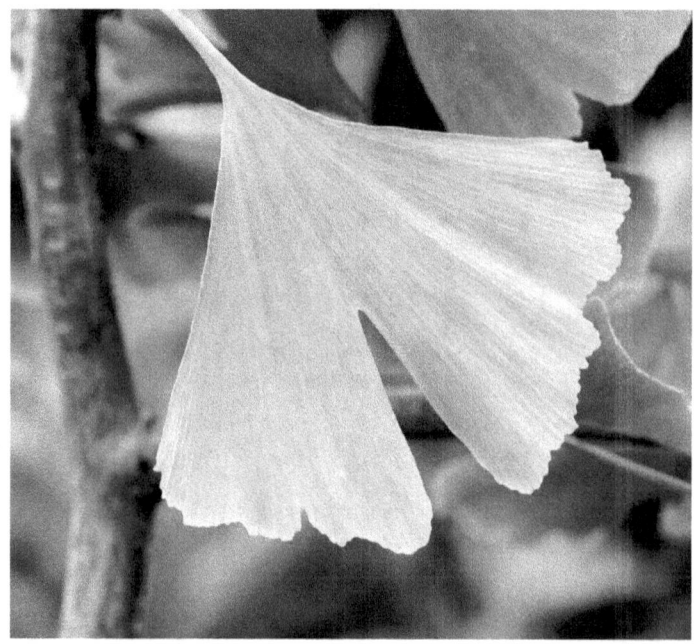

Ginkgo biloba calms anxiety without causing drowsiness, and prevents sleepiness in patients during the day when they take antiparkinsonian drugs.

It also improves memory and attention and, in experimental animals, acts as a neuroprotector in the nigrostriatal system. It increases blood flow with its antiplatelet effect, which should be considered when combining with aspirin or clopidogrel; it is contraindicated with anticoagulants.

Ginkgo biloba

Ginkgo relieves some symptoms of Parkinson's disease, is neuroprotective,[57,134,473] improves mental functions and increases cerebral blood flow.[547]

To mention another advantage, when taking *Ginkgo biloba* patients become alert and watchful, and the daytime sleepiness caused by antiparkinsonian drugs is avoided.[134,633]

Moreover, it calms the anxiety[378,598] which causes Parkinson's symptoms to get worse. If we eliminate anxiety, tremor decreases and mobility improves. This type of effect is desirable because we know that only symptomatic treatment of this disease is available, so it is best to ameliorate symptoms with minimal amounts of antiparkinsonian drugs. In addition, patients taking ginkgo seem to need fewer psychotropics.[19]

The neuroprotective effect is demonstrated in experimental animals. In mice with MPTP-induced parkinsonism, ginkgo prevents nigrostriatal neurodegeneracion. It is assumed that it may act by decreasing oxidative stress or by inhibiting MAO (monoamine oxidase enzyme).[9,467,468,547,587]

Some doctors say they do not prescribe *Gingko biloba* because they believe it is "like water", just a placebo. However ginkgo must have potency of some sort: it can cause bleeding in anticoagulated patients and fainting in hypotensive individuals; it may even lead to coma when combined with trazodone.[227]

Ginkgo biloba extract works as an antiaggregating agent, hence it facilitates bleeding and enhances the effects of aspirin,[54, 114] acts on the blood vessels (possibly producing blood pressure problems), and it influences the central nervous system (and may interact with antidepressants).[114]

FUNDAMENTALS

Ginkgo biloba leaves contain active substances that are very beneficial both separately and (especially) synergistically. Among the standardized extracts, EGb 761 (Tanakene) is the most notable with an appropriate content of 24% of flavonoids and 6% of terpenoids. When used correctly it is safe, increases cerebral blood flow, improves memory; it is an antioxidant,[57] protects rats with MPTP-induced parkinsonism[609] and benefits people with neuro-degenerative diseases such as Alzheimer and Parkinson.[57, 134, 473, 632, 633]

RELIEF OF ANXIETY

In elderly or cognitively impaired people, ginkgo relieves anxiety.[378, 598] It modulates the GABA systems (chemical messengers widely distributed in the brain) and reduces agitation, similar to benzodiazepines, although the exact mechanism is unknown.

INCREASE IN MEMORY AND ATTENTION

Ginkgo may, to some extent, improve memory and cognitive functions, including attention and mental processing speed. A nootropic effect can be objectified by electroencephalography.[164]

At the University of Bordeaux in France, 3,612 people over age 65 were selected; 589 were treated with ginkgo, 149 took piracetam and the remaining 2,874 took nothing. All were monitored for 20 years. At the end of this period, those treated with ginkgo maintained more memory than the others and, somewhat curiously, those who had been on piracetam performed worse than those who had taken nothing.[19]

IMPROVED COGNITION AND RELATIONSHIPS

In healthy young people, a single dose of ginkgo (300-400 mg) improves cognition and mood.[263] Ginkgo produces some benefit in dementia.[142.256] This is more evident when patients exhibit neuropsychiatric symptoms,[223, 256,397] even if they are severe.[289, 546]

There are many clinical human trials that do not meet the appropriate criteria or in which there is no reliable evidence.[49, 240, 570] However, in a recent meta-analysis of 298 human trials it was concluded that Ginkgo at doses of 240 mg/day is effective and safe in the treatment of dementia.[198]

In patients with mild to moderate Alzheimer's disease that were treated with ginkgo (160 mg/day) for 24 weeks, a cognitive improvement was found comparable to donepezil (5 mg), an anticholinesterase commonly prescribed for dementia.[354] In seven other studies in 410 patients with mild to moderate dementia (vascular or Alzheimer's), after 24 weeks, the ginkgo was safe and produced a significant improvement on the cognitive, psychopathological and functional levels, and in the quality of life of the patients and their caregivers.[205, 223, 224, 287, 288, 352, 398]

Ginkgo enhances cognitive ability in mice and improves dementia (scopolamine-induced), besides acting as anticholinesterase (such as donepezil and rivastigmine used for treating Alzheimer's patients).[109]

A LONGER LIFE

Those who take Ginkgo biloba are living longer according to a 13-year study of 3,500 people over 65 years.[107] The overall mortality rate was reduced by half. This seems far too optimistic but it has been demonstrated in small animals such as nematodes (*Canorhabditis elegans*)[601] and a few mammals.

DECREASED DYSKINESIAS

Dyskinesias were diminished after treatment with ginkgo in patients with abnormal movements caused by psychotropic drugs.[622]

BALANCE AND POSTURAL STABILITY

In disorders of balance and postural stability (from vestibular, vascular or undetermined origin), ginkgo (240 mg) was shown to be equally effective or more so than betahistine (32 mg) to relieve vertigo and dizziness, and is better tolerated.[527]

GINKGO IN PARKINSON'S DISEASE

Some have recommend ginkgo for treatment of Parkinson's and other neurodegenerative diseases.[111, 143, 378, 612] Anecdotally, one doctor has reported a dramatic improvement in his parkinsonian grandfather whom he prescribed ginkgo along with multivitamins.[102] Human trials are limited by methodological difficulties but there is experimental evidence in animal models in which parkinsonism has been induced (by injections of MPTP or 6-OHP).[9, 269, 467, 468, 547, 587, 609]

The extract of Ginkgo biloba (EGb 761) showed a neuro-protective effect in rats with experimental parkinsonism. The authors concluded that these data suggest a possible role for ginkgo in the treatment of Parkinson's disease.[5, 9, 269]

There is also another interesting aspect: in the rats treated with gingko, damage resulting from the levodopa therapy are lower; when administering levodopa some fresh injuries that occur are lesser if the levodopa is combined with ginkgo.[71]

MECHANISM

The mechanism behind the activity of Ginkgo biloba is complex and relates to its flavonoid, proanthocyanidin, and diterpene (ginkgolides A, B, C) content. This combination enhances cognitive processes, improves blood flow and tissue metabolism and prevents ischemia.

Ginkgo acts as an antioxidant, preventing deterioration of the hippocampus and improving neuronal plasticity;[111] it eliminates free radicals, especially nitric oxide[4, 42, 111] and inhibits platelet activating factor[526] which results in an anti-inflammatory effect.

Another mechanism of ginkgo activity is through the inhibition of MAO-B and COMT: it slows degradation of neurotransmitters such as dopamine, adrenaline and noradrenaline,[123, 547, 595, 600] decreases the action of glutamate, and also demonstrates GABA-ergic activity.[488]

SIDE EFFECTS

Ginkgo extract by mouth is well tolerated at the usual doses. It is a good idea to test its effect on blood pressure: sometimes it produces a slight rise that could be beneficial in some Parkinson's patients with usually low blood pressure.

Because of its antiplatelet effect, it should not be combined with anticoagulants: combined with warfarin it may cause bleeding. With other antiplatelets it is necessary to consider the synergistic effect (which sometimes is used therapeutically). In fact, combinations of aspirin and ginkgo are often used, as in a study in Taiwan.[88] When ginkgo has been associated with antiplatelets (and even anticoagulants) some authors consider that bleeding risk is negligible.[86]

Hemostasis (blood clotting) does not change significantly with ginkgo, and it has been suggested that safety is not affected when aspirin or warfarin are associated with it.[51] However, the possibility of idiosyncratic bleeding is not excluded and that combination should occur only under medical supervision. It is recommended that ginkgo be stopped two weeks before a planned surgery.[469]

As a precaution, patients should not mix ginkgo and trazodone (Deprax), although only one (dubious) relationship has been documented between this combination and a patient who experienced a coma.[168] Ginkgo may potentiate clonazepam (Rivotril) and modify the effects of alprazolam, antidepressants, anticonvulsants and other drugs that are metabolized via cytochrome. However, at recommended doses no significant disturbances have been disclosed.

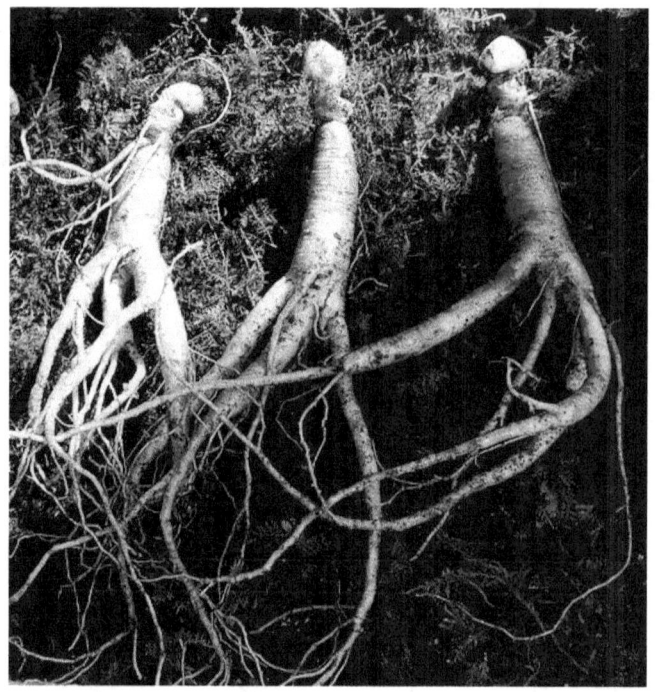

Ginseng may be useful to people with Parkinson's disease as a mental and physical activator.

It helps avoid the sleepiness caused by dopaminergic drugs, increases mental concentration and elevates mood and libido. It counteracts blood pressure drops and therefore should not be given to hypertensive or cardiac patients. It should not be mixed with anticoagulants or stimulants.

Ginseng

The wife of one of my Parkinson's patients once stated, "*I gave ginseng to Eduardo and he became very, very lively, but of course then I read the contraindications and I had to take it away; but in truth, it had been doing him good, he was a different man that day, with a strong will to do things; he was even walking better.*"

These words summarize what can be expected of ginseng in Parkinson's disease. It is a stimulant and a general activator, it elevates mood and libido, prevents daytime sleepiness, and compensates for the sudden drops in blood pressure that many Parkinson's patients tend to experience (due to the disease itself or to medication). But those benefits become inconveniences in very elderly patients or those with hypertension or heart disease.

Ginseng is a neuroprotector which can be considered in the treatment of Parkinson's[97, 174, 406] and other degenerative diseases of the nervous system such as Alzheimer's, Huntington's chorea, major depression, stroke, amyotrophic lateral sclerosis (also known as ALS, or Lou Gehrig's disease) and multiple sclerosis.[97, 406]

The ginseng on the market varies widely in quality and concentration.[197] Those who buy "ginseng" do not usually know what they are taking. Is it Chinese, Korean, or American ginseng? What proportion of ginsenosides does it contain? (If it contains under 24%, it does not work.) Does the product actually contain what is on the label? Does the label even clearly describe the components and concentrations? There is much confusion regarding the various types of ginseng and the proportions of their active ingredients.

FUNDAMENTALS

Five thousand years ago, Chinese Emperors took ginseng to sustain youth and promote energy and longevity. Ginseng grows in cold, mountainous areas of China, Korea, Siberia and Canada. Its medicinal root becomes more valuable with age because it accumulates ginsenosides, its pharmacologically active substances, with time.

Ginseng is the quintessential Asian tonic: it enhances physical performance without producing excitation,[81, 596, 597] it is an aphrodisiac, antioxidant, antidepressant, anxiolytic and nootropic agent; ginseng improves memory, strengthens arithmetic ability[447] and overall mental activity.[406]

It is recommended against aging as well as Parkinson's, and other neuro-degenerative diseases.[116, 502] In combination with Ginkgo biloba, it has been used in children with attention deficit hyperactivity disorder.[201] Its efficacy as a nootropic (a substance that supports memory and general mental activity) is associated with the moderation of anxiety.[100]

At the beginning of treatment, ginseng is taken in repeated doses that are later diminished as the desired effects are achieved, arriving at a maintenance dose for a period of three months. Dosage-free intervals between treatments are recommended.

VARIETIES OF GINSENG

The name ginseng is given to numerous species of plants of the genus *Panax* (meaning 'panacea' in Latin) and others which are not ginseng but have similar properties. The one that is commonly known as ginseng is the species *Panax ginseng* or Asian ginseng (Chinese or Korean), which is the most potent variety, the most widely used for medical purposes, and which contains the most active substances.

Ginsenosides make up over 20 varieties of saponins (triterpenoid glycosides). Two groups are distinguished: RB-1 (with sedative and analgesic properties) and RG-1 (with stimulant, anti-fatigue and vasodilatory actions). Ginsenosides Rg1 and Rb1 have neurotrophic and neuroprotective effects, which improve mood and cognitive functions,[263, 479, 493] mental health and quality of life.[140]

Furthermore, there are the American variety (*Panax quinquefolium L.*) and Russian or Siberian ginseng (*Eleutherococcus senticosus Maxim.*), containing ginsenosides in various proportions producing somewhat different effects. In simpler terms, we could say that the Asian (*Panax ginseng*, rich in Rg1, Rb2 and Rc) has stronger boosting effect on brain activity while they are attributed greater antineoplastic possibilities as opposed to American ginseng (*Panax quinquefolium*, with predominance of Rb1, Re and Rd).[93]

HUMAN TRIALS

Human trials are very heterogeneous because different types of ginseng are conflated. Moreover, there are variations in the manner in which the plants are cultivated, in their genetic origin, and their age (older specimens are richer in ginsenosides). Moreover, as true ginseng root is very expensive, adulterations are common. All this contributes to highly variable results in the studies carried out in humans.

There is another factor that determines erratic results: ginsenosides are largely metabolized by the intestinal microflora and some of its derivatives are also active. Therefore each individual responds differently to ginseng depending on the composition of his or her intestinal flora.

ANIMAL MODELS OF PARKINSON'S DISEASE

In rats with 6-OHP-induced parkinsonism, the pseudo-ginsenoside f11 improved locomotion, balance and coordination, being considered a neuroprotector.[584] In rodents with MPTP-induced parkinsonism, oral administration of ginseng prevents locomotor dysfunction,[571] improves behavioral disorders and reduces death of dopaminergic neurons.[248, 317]

Ginsenoside Rg1 specifically has been demonstrated as a neuroprotective and immunomodulator agent and represents promise for treating Parkinson's disease; it produces motor improvement,[241] reduces the loss of dopaminergic neurons and mediates in central and peripheral inflammation.[95, 624, 625]

Ginseng reduced the loss of dopaminergic cells, microgliosis and synuclein accumulation in rodents with both MPTP-induced parkinsonism, and in a new animal model of progressive parkinsonism produced with a special diet (BSSG, chronic dietary phytosterol glucoside).[571, 572]

COGNITIVE IMPROVEMENT

Ginseng extracts stimulate mental activity and concentration, and improve cognitive functions in patients with moderate to severe Alzheimer's disease.[203, 268] When standardized *Panax ginseng* extract (G115: Pharmaton) is given to rats their memory, learning, physical and locomotor ability are increased (using maze tests).[427]

In animals, ginseng modulates cholinergic receptors,[99, 482] improves visual memory[100] and increases cerebral flow.[265] It acts as a neurotrophic and neuroprotective factor in the hippocampus[270,296] and cerebral cortex[375], removes free radicals[271] and enhances immunity.[507]

ADAPTOGEN

Ginseng is also a good adaptogen: it can prevent damage by stress. In rats subjected to chronic stress, corticoid plasma levels rise while dopamine and serotonin in the hippocampus and cerebral cortex are decreased. These changes are prevented by ginseng (*Panax quinquefolium*).[503]

APHRODISIAC

Ginseng acts as an aphrodisiac by increasing libido and copulatory capacity when consumed.[212,390,485] Ginsenosides facilitate erection by vasodilation of the corpus cavernosum[485] and facilitate copulatory behavior by releasing hormones and catecholamines in the hypothalamus.[390]

MECHANISM OF ACTION

The major neuroprotective ginsenosides are Rn1, Rg1, Rd and Re, which inhibit neuroinflammation and oxidative stress. They act as immunomodulators, decrease toxin-induced apoptosis, lower iron levels in the substantia nigra, and regulate the activity of NMDA receptors.

Ginsenosides also act on the brain by other mechanisms including glutamate and monoamine transmission, the production of nitric oxide, formation of beta-amyloid, tau phosphorylation, and pathways of cellular stress, neuronal survival, apoptosis, neurodegeneration, microglia, astrocytes, oligodendrocytes and cerebral microvasculature.[174, 406]

SIDE EFFECTS

Insomnia is the most common side effect of ginseng. It can also cause agitation, some mild gastrointestinal discomfort and prolonged erection. Avoid mixing ginseng with caffeine or other stimulants (ephedrine and the like) or with drugs that alter heart rate. It may interact with warfarin, phenelzine and alcohol[101] and *some* manic episodes have been described.[141, 573]

Ginseng is contraindicated in patients receiving anticoagulants and will be used with caution in those taking antiplatelet agents. It should be avoided by people with agitation or a history of schizophrenia or cardiovascular disorders. It has a hypoglycemic effect, which must be taken into account in diabetics under treatment. Ginseng should be administered in limited periods (six months or less).

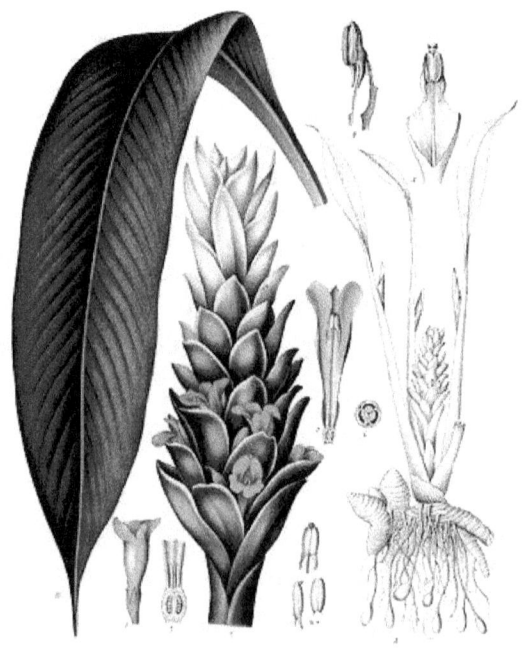

Turmeric opens new horizons for the treatment of Parkinson's and other neurodegenerative diseases. It is another research pathway.

It activates multifactorial mechanisms, including changes in expression of genes related to aging. In experimental animals it lengthens life and shows neuroprotective capacity. It also has antidepressant effects comparable to fluoxetine.

Turmeric

The yellow color in curry is due to turmeric, a novel treatment for Parkinson's disease that will be important in the future because it acts through a unique mechanism.

Up to now, the main therapy for Parkinson's was to replace dopamine. Turmeric acts by other routes: it improves the response of age-related genes[505] resulting in a longer and healthier lifespan in laboratory animals.

Curcumin, one of its ingredients, is an antioxidant which inhibits MAO-B and slows the accumulation of alpha-synuclein: and this is the basis for its utility in treating Parkinson's disease.[238]

Human studies are still scarce, but the experimental evidence *in vitro* and in animal models leaves no doubt of its viability. Fruit flies (*Drosophila*) live longer and healthier when given curcumin, a polyphenol that acts on their genes and/or the way they are expressed, in other words, a genotropic drug.[296] The same applies when mice or nematodes are fed with curcumin: they live longer,[505] though this may sound like science fiction.

Curcumin also protects the animals with toxin-induced parkinsonism. These rats and flies fed with curcumin suffer fewer injuries in dopaminergic neurons and display fewer motor or behavioral disorders. Rats and flies fed with curcumin experience fewer lesions in dopaminergic neurons and fewer movement and behavioral disorders.[233, 329, 393, 446, 616]

In patients, turmeric relieves depression as much as fluoxetine,[486] improves cognition and relieves the poor intestinal motility that so compromises Parkinson's patients.

Turmeric in the diet produces prolonged benefits and is safe: no studies in humans or animals have found toxic effects.[245, 284]

FUNDAMENTALS

The roots of Curcuma longa contain curcumin, a polyphenol that is neuroprotective in Parkinson's, Alzheimer's and other neurodegenerative diseases.[392, 623]

Curcumin modulates the expression of age-related genes, acts as an anti-oxidant and anti-inflammatory agent, inhibits MAO[238], prevents the accumulation of alpha-synuclein and regulates other molecular targets,[623] thereby opening new therapeutic horizons.[297, 392, 531] Despite its limited bioavailability[108] it results effective with the substances in which it breaks down.[504]

ANIMALS WITH PARKINSONISM

Rodents with MPTP-induced parkinsonism previously fed with turmeric remain "protected", and that mitigates the damage of nigrostriatal neurons and their associated symptoms.[233, 393, 616]

In rats with 6-OHDA-induced parkinsonism, curcumin reversed anhedonia and improved behavior, increased neurotransmitters such as dopamine, regenerated damage to the hippocampus[530, 606] and protected dopaminergic nigrostriatal neurons.[131, 561, 562, 618] Curcumin also prevents motor disorders and neuronal damage in mice with parkinsonism induced by MPTP[393] or intracerebral homocysteine.[329] That benefit of turmeric has also been shown in other animal models of parkinsonism. In Drosophila flies, motor symptoms are delayed, oxidative stress and apoptosis are reduced, and their lifespans are prolonged.[518]

Curcumin, is "genotropic", i.e. it modifies genes or the manner in which they are expressed, according to their growth stage. Thus, in Drosophila flies with Paraquat-induced parkinsonism, curcumin prevents motor disorders if applied when they are in the earlier stages, but not later.[428]

SYNUCLEIN ACCUMULATION IN THE BRAIN

Neurodegeneration in mice may also be genetically induced resulting in brain accumulation of synuclein and motor disorders resembling parkinsonism. However, acute or chronic treatment with curcumin limits the deposit of that protein and a clear improvement in motor disorders is observed.[532]

MEMORY RECOVERY IN OLDER MICE

In a model of cognitive impairment in mice (induced by subcutaneous D-galactose) curcumin improved learning and spatial memory.[396]

In old mice with memory deficits, after taking curcumin for three weeks, a significant improvement was observed. It was deduced that this would relate, at least in part, to the activation of neuronal nitric oxide in certain brain regions. This suggests the potential of curcumin as a preventive of general cognitive impairment.

ANTIDEPRESSANT

In humans turmeric is a good antidepressant, as effective as fluoxetine.[486] In 60 patients diagnosed with major depressive disorder the response to fluoxetine (20 mg), curcumin (1000 mg) or combination of them was evaluated. After 6 weeks all three groups improved with similar results between the pharmaceutical (64.7%) and curcumin (62.5%), and even more so when given together (77.8%).[486] The antidepressant efficacy of turmeric is endorsed in bibliographic meta-analysis.[17]

An antidepressant action has also been proven in rodents. In an animal model of chronic mild stress when turmeric was administered to male rats the expected alteration of the hypothalamic-pituitary-adrenal were decreased.[603]

Two separate studies[279, 602] with mice subjected to a forced swim test coincide in results and conclusions: when animals were fed with turmeric extract for three weeks there was decreased neurochemical (decreased serotonin, dopamine and norepinephrine) and neuroendocrine (elevated cortisol and ACTH-RF) dysregulation, and animals did not lack mobility as expected. [279, 602]

MECHANISM OF ACTION

Researchers agree that curcumin is neuroprotective but invokes different mechanisms including the modulation of mitochondrial dysfunction and glutathione metabolism,[229] a chelating action of iron suppressing the degeneration of neurons in the substantia nigra,[131] inhibition of Jun-kinase pathways to prevent cell death[616] or by opposing aggregation of alpha-synuclein.[8, 239, 549]

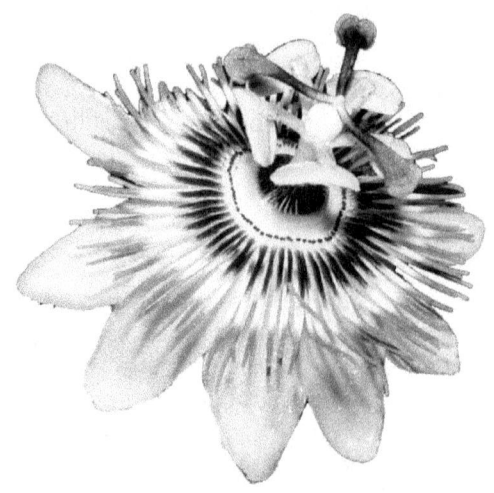

Passionflower improves tremor without the problems caused by anticholinergics and relieves anxiety and insomnia without the side effects of benzodiazepines.

These characteristics make this substance potentially useful to many people with Parkinson's disease.

Passiflora

Passiflora, known also as the passionflower, is very useful in Parkinson's disease. It improves tremor, avoiding usual side effects of anticholinergic medication, and relieves anxiety and insomnia without the undesireable effects of the use of benzodiazepines.

Treatment of tremor is difficult. Levodopa and dopamine clearly improve general hypokinesias and bradykinesia but its effect on tremor is limited.

In young people without cognitive impairment an anticholinergic can be used, but in patients over 60 years, complications are frequent: memory impairment, hallucinations and others (dry mouth, increased constipation, glaucoma, etc.)

Passiflora directly improves tremor, and also relieves anxiety and insomnia, other common Parkinson's symptoms, so treatment with benzodiazepines can be substituted, thus avoiding impairment of memory and balance.

It is also antispasmodic (relieves intestinal spams) and contributes to reducing blood pressure. In addition, it alleviates muscular cramps and calms the sympathetic nervous system, so easily excited in parkinsonism.

Passiflora should be taken under medical supervision because, although it has few side effects, it is an effective sedative that may interact with other tranquilizers.

FUNDAMENTALS

Passiflora, or the passion flower plant, is a climbing vine with large red flowers (Passiflora incarnata). Its active ingredient, pasiflorina, structurally resembles morphine but is not addictive.

It is a popular remedy for insomnia and nervousness and relieves cough.[118, 119, 120, 487] *Passiflora incarnata* is preferably used, a variety not to be confused with *Passiflora edulis* (edible).

ANXIOLYTIC AND SEDATIVE QUALITIES

Currently passionflower is considered a reliable anxiolytic and sedative[121, 278, 281, 533] as effective as oxazepam and causing less functional impairment.[13] Therefore it is useful for parkinsonian symptoms in which walking is affected by benzodiazepine treatments.

While preparing for surgery[384] and epidural anesthesia, passionflower by mouth suppresses anxiety without inducing psychomotor or hemodynamic changes.[30] In another study, 40 people from 18-35 years had a cup of passiflora infusion for 7 days and their quality of sleep was subjectively improved.[401]

Anxiety and stress were decreased in rats when passiflora was added to their drinking water. Spatial memory was also improved and a reduction in glutamic acid (in the hippocampus) and serotonin (in the cerebral cortex) were observed.

MECHANISM OF ACTION

Passiflora acts through facilitation of GABA (gamma-amino butyric acid) -receptors.[25, 234]

An anxiolytic effect of passionflower (375 mg / kg) comparable to diazepam (1.5 mg / kg) has been described in mice. This anxiolytic activity is mediated by GABA as has been demonstrated *in vivo*.[187, 188] In rats an extract of Passiflora (chrysin 2 mg / kg) was similar to midazolam (2 mg / kg) but with a smaller anxiolytic effect.

NEUROPROTECTIVE AND ANTICONVULSANT QUALITIES

Passiflora suppresses pentilenefetrazol-induced convulsions in mice[309, 520] and improves postictal depression (unlike diazepam, which worsens it).[520]

ANALGESIC AND OTHER EFFECTS

Pain is common with Parkinson's. Passiflora relieves pain and cough: it is considered a "soft morphine" and non-addictive.[118, 119, 121] Indeed, it is used as a remedy against withdrawal syndrome when narcotics, benzo-diazepines or cannabis are being withdrawn.[12, 117, 122]

Benzoflavone, one of its components, is an aphrodisiac and prevents sexual decline in older male rats.[117]

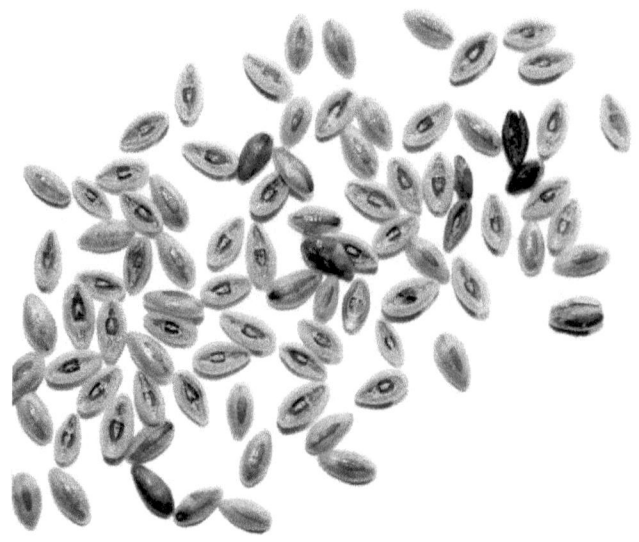

Plantago ovata seeds increase gastrointestinal motility resulting in a more efficient and stable absorption of levodopa, and that leads to a clear improvement of parkinsonian symptoms.

Plantago ovata

Constipation begins before tremor and rigidity, and then gradually becomes more and more troublesome as Parkinson's disease progresses. When the stomach is slow to empty, levodopa is not well absorbed. This is why *Plantago ovata* is important: when the bowel is moving, everything works better. Plantago husks improve and increase gastrointestinal motility;[39] more bowel movement means a higher amount of levodopa is absorbed, resulting in a greater improvement of symptoms.[29, 31]

When patients see their symptoms worsen they may change their medication and even consult another neurologist trying to find relief. In some cases the problem may not be ineffective medication, but rather that the pills are not processed due to slow gastrointestinal movement. The solution is simple: to use a natural laxative like *Plantago ovata*.

FUNDAMENTALS

In a study with rabbits which were administered levodopa in isolation[170] and later with carbidopa,[150] those that were given an additional dose of *Plantago ovata* husks were found to experience more efficient absorption of levodopa, and the maximum initial peak was descreased; after a period of time, the group taking the husk reported higher and more stable concentrations of levodopa at any given time. Eighteen patients taking levodopa/carbidopa were given either Plantago or a placebo for 35 days. Those who took Plantago had decreased plasmatic peaks of levodopa, and the levels were much more stable, resulting in a greater clinical benefit.[152] Such improvement in levodopa kinetics could also be useful even for Parkinson's patients without constipation.

In another study with 79 patients it has been shown that after using maintenance laxatives, rigidity is improved. That suggests there may be a gastrointestinal disorder in the pathogenesis of Parkinson's disease: intestinal dysbiosis causes decreased bowel mobility and this could favor deposition of abnormal proteins.[32]

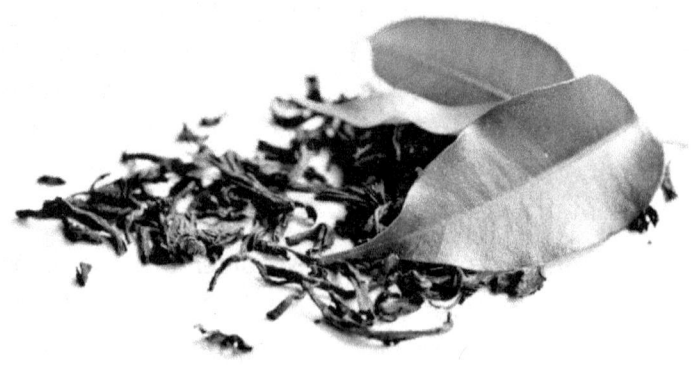

People who regularly drink **tea** are less likely to suffer from Parkinson's disease. In patients, green tea increases the effect of antiparkinsonian drugs because it contains poly-phenols which are neuroprotective and act in a way similar to carbidopa, entacapone and rasagiline.

In addition, it provides theine (which increases mental alertness) and theophylline (which improves tremor and motor capacity).

).

Green tea

A cup of green tea contains substances with effects similar to those of carbidopa, entacapone and rasagiline. Patients should be aware that green tea increases the effect of levodopa and other dopaminergic drugs. On the other hand, or perhaps related to this, those who drink tea have about half the chance of suffering from Parkinson's disease.

Each cup of tea contains, depending on the variety, 10 to 80 mg of **theine**, an alkaloid equivalent to caffeine with a somewhat more lasting effect. Drinking tea increases mental alertness, and shortens reaction time.[135, 207, 232, 305] Tea, especially green tea, also contains other beneficial substances: theophylline and polyphenols.

Theophylline, an adenosine antagonist, improves tremor and motor ability in patients, and enhances the effects of levodopa.

Polyphenols are antioxidant and neuroprotective, and somehow prevent cell damage due to aging. In addition, they have effects similar to carbidopa (Sinemet) or benserazide (Madopar), and others that work in a similar way to entacapone (Comtan, Stalevo) or selegiline (Eldepryl) and rasagiline (Azilect).

All these drugs increase the effectiveness of levodopa because they slow the enzymes that destroy (metabolise) it: they inhibit decarboxylase, COMT (catechol-ortho-methyl transferase) and MAO-B (mono-amino oxidase B).

Green tea (a source of polyphenols) does the same, and when taken with levodopa and other dopaminergic drugs, enhances its effect.[136] That capacity must be taken into account in order both to take advantage of the benefits and to prevent overdose. Green tea also enhances the natural levodopa of mucuna as we have observed in one patient[179, 180](see the chapter about mucuna).

Polyphenols contained in green tea have demonstrated neuroprotective effectiveness in animals and cell cultures, and possibly protect against Parkinson's and other neurodegenerative diseases.[416]

FUNDAMENTALS

Disregarding water, tea is the most consumed beverage in the world. There are several types of tea depending on which part of the plant (*Camellia sinensis*) is used and its preparation. Green tea does not go through the transformation process (in which the leaves are steamed and then dried), and it contains less theine.

Black tea leaves are fermented and darkened and sometimes flavored with wood, nuts, flowers (jasmine) or essences (bergamot in *Earl Grey*), and contain more theine. The *Oolong* variety is only partially fermented. White tea is obtained from buds and young leaves, and then thoroughly dried.

Tea (green or black) is neuroprotective. Drinking two cups of tea a day will cut the risk of acquiring Parkinson's by half.[23, 41, 87, 91, 235, 474, 475] Parkinson's disease is less prevalent in regions where tea is regularly consumed.[416] Green tea could prevent Parkinson's disease and even slow its evolution once it is established, although the mechanisms are not entirely understood.[79, 251, 326]

THEINE

Theine is the caffeine found in tea. Actually it is essentially the same substance as caffein, an alkaloid, but theine is absorbed more slowly due to the polyphenols contained in the tea. This avoids the "peak" effect (i.e., the rapid rise in stimulation that occurs with coffee), resulting in a more consistent and prolonged effect of arousal when tea is consumed.

THEOPHYLLINE

Theophylline is an antagonist of adenosine receptors (A2a) that improves tremor and motor ability in patients,[328] extending its *on* (low symptom) period.[276] Therefore it has been proposed as a routine treatment for Parkinson's disease.[327, 328]

When adenosine A2a receptors are blocked in experimental animals, levodopa is enhanced.

In one study,[38] 15 patients with moderate / advanced Parkinson's disease were treated with low doses of levodopa combined with KW-6002 (A-2A selective antagonist of adenosine). Its effects were enhanced (36% more than with levodopa alone), and fewer dyskinesias were observed. All symptoms improved, especially resting tremor.[38]

POLYPHENOLS

Tea polyphenols are potent antioxidants, which slow the aging process and protect neurons against Parkinson's and Alzheimer's disease.[415, 416, 590] The primary one, epigalocatecín-gallate, reduces the production of beta-amyloid[300], and also acts as an anti-oxidant, iron chelator and apoptosis inhibitor.[10, 301, 302, 303, 589]

ENHANCEMENT OF LEVODOPA WITH POLYPHENOLS AND THEOPHYLLINE

Levodopa is no longer prescribed in isolation. When levodopa reaches the bloodstream, it comes into contact with decarboxylase, an enzyme that quickly metabolizes it into dopamine, eradicating it before it reaches the brain. For this reason, levodopa is commercially available in combination with a decarboxylase inhibitor: carbidopa (Sinemet) or benserazide (Madopar).

Several green tea polyphenols (epicatechin and epicatechin-gallate) produce a similar effect by inhibiting decarboxylase[47, 379, 449] and, perhaps more specifically, resulting in a more beneficial treatment with levodopa.[379]

In 84 adults with Down syndrome after taking green tea extract for a year, various cognitive functions were improved: including visual recognition memory, inhibitory control and adaptive behavior.[112] Tea consumption also reduces the risk of dementia and cognitive impairment.[608]

EXPERIMENTAL ANIMALS AND CELL CULTURES

In mice with MPTP-induced parkinsonism green tea (with high levels of epicatechin-gallate) prevents neurochemical alterations of the *substantia nigra*.[98, 186, 402, 415, 613]

There is a transgenic model of parkinsonism in fruit flies in which synuclein accumulates in the brain, with loss of dopaminergic neurons, causing decrease of mobility and the ability to jump. That effect is delayed if their diet is supplemented with epicatechin, a component of green tea.[517]

In cell cultures, extracts of green tea and black tea decrease hydroxydopamine-induced toxicity.[300, 302, 589] Green tea polyphenols also protect dopaminergic neurons because they inhibit oxidation processes and block some pathways of nitrous oxide (NO) .[191]

MECHANISM OF ACTION

Tea prevents death from many causes, including cardiovascular complications.[323, 324, 325, 326] Catechins and other components of tea have many useful properties, especially for the elderly, and even more so for Parkinson's patients taking levodopa.

These components of green tea act as natural inhibitors of MAO (which increases with age and promotes neurodegeneration), COMT (which methylate levodopa) and decarboxylase (which rapidly removes levodopa from the bloodstream). By inhibiting these three enzymes tea improves the availability of levodopa and dopamine.

In patients treated with levodopa and carbidopa, epigallocatechin gallate (contained in tea) seems beneficial, as deduced from studies in rats and in cell cultures. Gallate epigallocatechin, the main tea polyphenol, restrains methylation of levodopa (and therefore slows its elimination from the bloodstream) and, additionally, it protects the hippocampus from oxidative neurodegeneration.[254, 255] Quercetin, a tea flavonoid, produces a similar effect by inhibiting COMT.[255]

The enzyme mono-amino oxidase (MAO), increases with age and contributes to the degeneration of the central nervous system, decreasing dopamine in the brain. In an attempt to inhibit the MAO enzyme, Eldepryl (selegiline) or Azilect (rasagiline) are given to Parkinson's patients, especially at the onset of the disease, thereby evoking its neuroprotective effect.

As we can see, there are natural neuroprotectors which inhibit MAO, and are found in tea and other products such as turmeric.[355] They are beneficial for older people and particularly for patients with Parkinson disease.

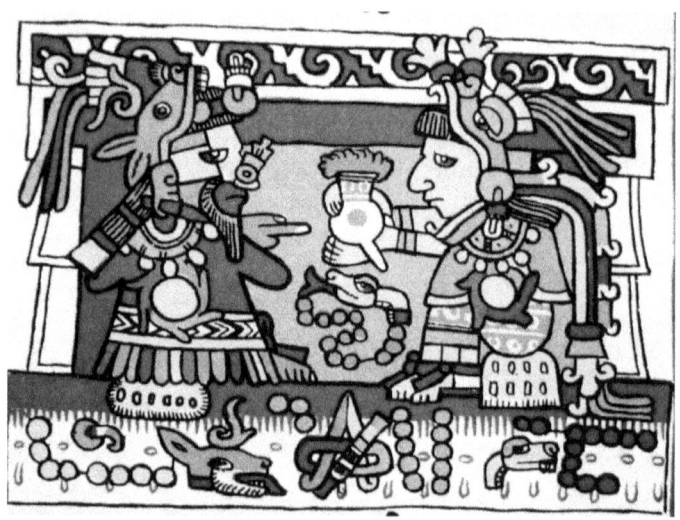

Montezuma sharing a chocolate beverage

Chocolate provides nutrients (flavonoids) and psycho-active substances (theobromine, fenietilamina). It also induces feelings of "reward" and pleasure with its taste, texture and aroma, thereby activating dopaminergic systems, releasing endorphins and improving mood. Parkinson's patients frequently eat chocolate. Caution should be observed for those treated with MAO inhibitors.

Cacao (Chocolate)

Patients with Parkinson's or depression tend to eat a lot of chocolate, perhaps because they sense that they need it. Chocolate contains many biogenic amines acting as antiparkinsonian drugs.[599]

Chocolate contains phenylethylamine which increases dopamine, but little of this reaches the brain because it is eliminated from the bloodstream by the enzyme monoamine oxidase.

What happens when a Parkinson's patient treated with Azilect or Eldepryl (which inhibits that enzyme) eats chocolate? Probably a larger amount of phenylethylamine will reach the brain causing a sense of euphoria.

Chocolate provides calories, supplies nutrients (polyphenols) and also nourishes emotionally (see chapter on "Sensory Diet"): the taste and texture of a chocolate treat, the feeling of luxury that it transmits, the pleasure, this nourishes us emotionally: it's a food for our senses, a hedonic (pleasure-based) reward, which provides wellness and releases endorphins (our inner morphine).

In the 1980s the "chocolate theory of love", suggesting that phenylethylamine produces a feeling of happiness as infatuation, became widespread. It was actually an urban legend, but chocolate has something: is the food that most changes mood. Its psychoactive components, anandamide, caffeine, phenylethanolamine and magnesium, generate pleasure.[576] People tend to eat chocolate when they feel down.[44]

FUNDAMENTALS

Two thousand years ago the Maya and Aztec people obtained chocolate from cocoa. They ground the grains, and then boiled them and mixed them with cornmeal, spices or honey, to make *xocolatl* a strong-tasting beverage that provided a great amount of energy and vitality.

Chocolate acts as an anti-inflammatory, a neuroprotector and a cardioprotective agent, and it increases the bioavailability of nitrous oxide thus improving arterial pressure, platelet function and blood flow.[576]

NUTRIENTS AND ACTIVE SUBSTANCES

Chocolate is a valuable source of quickly available energy, and is rich in carbohydrates, fats, proteins, vitamins and trace elements. It also contains flavonoids, methylxanthines (caffeine, theophylline, theobromine), biogenic amines (phenylethylamine, histamine, tyramine) and fatty acids; the latter act in a fashion similar to cannabis because they inhibit the elimination of our natural endocannabinoids.[63, 567, 576]

FLAVONOIDS

Cocoa flavonoids have high antioxidant activity and are beneficial against neurodegenerative and cardiovascular diseases.[499, 538] When mixed with milk, absorption decreases, so dark chocolate is preferable.[498]

THEOBROMINE

The main alkaloid found in cocoa and chocolate is theobromine, which has a minor "perk up" effect in comparison to caffeine.[247] In mice a theobromine-enriched diet increases levels of dopamine, acetylcholine and norepinephrine, which benefits the "cognitive reserve".[151] An anti-inflammatory and anti-tumor effect is also attributed to it.[542]

PHENYLETHYLAMINE

Phenylethylamine increases dopamine levels in the brain by releasing substances that improve mood, balance blood pressure, elevate heart rate and increase sexual appetite.

However only some chocolates contain phenylethylamine, and it reaches the brain in small quantities. Chocolate biogenic amines may provide a different benefit: stimulation of the gut and enhancing of gastrointestinal circulation[58] ... which would increase the absorption of levodopa.

SALSOLINOL

Chocolate may owe its addictive quality to salsolinol, a D2-D3 dopaminergic substance, which is one of its main psychoactive components.[365] Salsolinol is also produced by the body. Its elimination by urine is low in Parkinson's patients and increases when they are treated with levodopa.[577]

CHOCOLATE AS A DRUG

Chocolate has some characteristics of mind-altering drugs and in susceptible people it may trigger psycho-pharmacological reactions, affective disorders and addictive behaviors similar to alcoholism, drug abuse or sex addiction.[63, 565]

Apart from its psychoactive components chocolate, like all pleasant food, generates endorphins.[44, 320, 367, 407, 576] Motivation is induced sensorially.[477] This is why cocoa capsules barely have any effect: the "reward" obtained is not sufficient.[367]

CHOCOLATE AND MOOD

There are people who crave chocolate and take it unaware that they are "self-medicating" to compensate for deficiencies in their diet (e.g. magnesium) or to balance out low levels of certain neurotransmitters (serotonin and dopamine) that regulate mood, appetite and compulsive behaviors. [377]

Depression increases one's appetite for chocolate and other sweet rewards.[593] The desire to eat chocolate is usually episodic and changes according to hormonal modifications; women often eat more of it just before menstruation [63, 368] and cravings for it decrease after menopause.[423]

ADDICTION, SELF-INDULGENCE AND PARKINSON'S DISEASE

Dependence on chocolate is reminiscent of that of nicotine and other drugs, leading to activation of the pre-frontal cortex. [494] Rehabilitated alcoholics often (78%) transfer their addiction to chocolate, coffee, tobacco and other substances that stimulate neural systems of reward and pleasure.[250]

There is debate as to the existence of addictive personalities and their relationship to the level of dopamine in the brain,[478] but it is known that there is less risk of Parkinson's disease among those who have a tendency to use recreational drugs.

Chocolate can be a suitable "soft drug" for Parkinson's patients: it is a luxury for the senses and a little sinful, affording them a small visual, sensory —and tasty— reward (provided neither diabetes nor obesity is an issue). It makes us feel good and activates our pleasure centers in the brain. The behavioral aspect of this response may be due to innate or acquired responses, or it may reflect anticipations or expectations (desire) based on our previous experiences of emotional reward.[409]

Furthermore, as Sinemet or Madopar are absorbed faster when mixed with carbohydrates, sometimes motor improvement occurs sooner when the tablet is paired with a chocolate candy.

EFFECT OF CHOCOLATE ON SLOWING COGNITIVE DECLINE

Eating chocolate reduces the risk of cognitive impairment.[380] In a study of 531 people over 65 years, controlled for four years, cognitive decline was lower among those who ate chocolate regularly.[380]

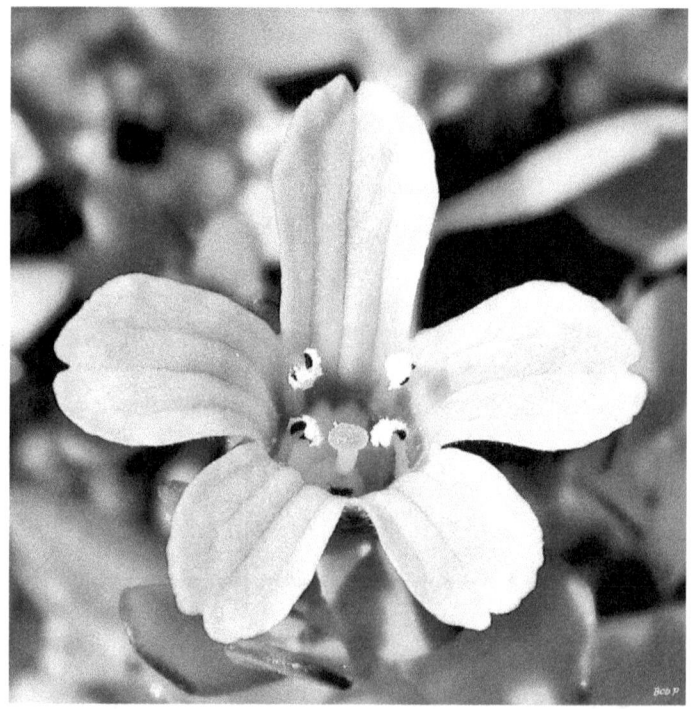

Bacopa strengthens memory and other cognitive functions both in humans and animals. It acts like the acetylcholinesterase inhibitors used in dementias and MAO inhibitors that are prescribed in Parkinson's disease.

In animal models of parkinsonism bacopa protects dopaminergic neurons from toxic injuries and prevents trembling and lack of mobility.

Bacopa

Bacopa extract is an antidote to parkinsonism in experimental animals, protecting them from tremor and hypokinesias, which are produced by toxins.

Bacopa monnieri ('Brahmi') is one of the main natural remedies to enhance memory and other cognitive functions, it acts as a neuroprotector and a neural tonic. Tests indicate its potential in treating Parkinson's disease, Alzheimer's and other types of neurodegeneration.[2, 342, 421]

In addition to its effects as a cerebral stimulant (it is considered a nerve tonic and memory enhancer in Ayurveda) Bacopa is a great "adaptogen": it protects against the effects of acute and chronic stress. Stress facilitates the appearance and development of neurodegenerative disorders (Parkinson's included).[177]

FUNDAMENTALS

Bacopa has proved its neuroprotective properties in animal models of Parkinson's, dementia and stress, and in humans it has shown some cognitive benefits.

CLINICAL TRIALS

There are several controlled trials with humans demonstrating that Bacopa and its components are nootropics (they promote brain function) and potentially improve patients with dementia, Parkinson's and epilepsy.[2]

In other randomized, controlled, double-blind studies, Bacopa significantly improved memory in 98 healthy people over 55 years of age.[382] A study of 60 healthy subjects (mean age 62 years) treated with Bacopa extract (300 and 600 mg daily), or a placebo, for 12 weeks, showed improvement in working memory and decreased latencies of N100 and P300 waves for elicited event-related potential. This means that reaction time to an event is reduced. Additionally, an anticholinesterase action was observed (similar to the drugs used against Alzheimer's).[426]

ANIMALS WITH INDUCED PARKINSONISM

Studies in animals or cell cultures are more numerous. It has been shown that Bacopa strengthens brain capabilities by taking on various neuroprotective roles: as an antioxidant, by reducing the accumulation of beta-amyloid, increasing cerebral blood flow, inhibiting acetyl-cholinesterase and modulating various neurotransmitters (acetylcholine, serotonin and dopamina).[2, 109, 445]

In rats with 6-OHDA-induced parkinsonism, when they were previously treated over three weeks with Bacopa extract (20 and 40 mg / kg) there was a decrease of lesions in the striatum, and neurochemical alterations, and motor and behavioral disorders were disminished.[513]

In prepubertal mice with rotetone-induced parkinsonim when Bacopa is administered as a preventive therapy, it reduces oxidative damage and prevents striatal dopamine depletion.

The authors suggest that Bacopa would be effective in preventing and treating Parkinson's and other neurodegenerative diseases related to oxidative stress.[508]   The same favorable results from treatment with Bacopa were observed in fruit flies with rotetone-induced parkinsonism.[215]

In fruit flies with a genetic-induced parkinsonism (promoting synuclein accumulation in the brain) treatment with Bacopa significantly improved their mobility, increasing the insects' ability to jump.[230]

In a similar genetic model in nematodes (*Caernohabditis elegans*) Bacopa reduced the accumulation of alpha-synuclein and dopaminergic neuro-degeneration, thus it was concluded that it is a possible antiparkinson treatment.[228]

Comparable results were found in mice with Paraquat-induced parkinsonism: oral administration of Bacopa extract prevents injuries and symptoms that Paraquat normally produces, as well as decreasing striatal dopamine levels.[214]

ANIMALS WITH DEMENTIA

In male mice with scopolamine-induced "dementia" Bacopa extract produced clear cognitive improvement and decreased anticholinesterase activity (similar to Alzheimer's drugs).[109]

Other *in vitro* studies demonstrate that some components of Bacopa (bacopasides I and II) are MAO inhibitors which would support the claim that they have antiparkinson effects.[521]

In mice it has been shown that the extract of Bacopa enhances cognitive ability and improves dementia (induced with scopolamine), besides acting as an anticholinesterase such as donepezil and rivastigmine (used for treating Alzheimer's patients).[109]

In a model of reserpine-induced depression in mice, bacoside I (a component of Bacopa) showed an antidepressant effect, decreasing the lag time between immobility and behavioral changes.[309]

ANIMALS WITH STRESS

In rats undergoing acute and chronic stress a variety of damage and lesions occur: gastric ulcers; increased levels of glycemia, aminotransferase and creatine kinase; in addition to decreased spleen volume and enlarged adrenal glands. However, when they are previously treated with Bacopa (40-80 mg / kg), animals are protected, avoiding many of the injuries resulting from stress.[439]

In another test in rats subjected to chronic stress, steroid concentrations in plasma were high, while dopamine and serotonin were decreased in the hippocampus and the cortex. However these changes were prevented by treatment with brahmi (40 and 80 mg / kg). It follows that the Bacopa is a good adaptogen, capable of preventing damage by stress.[503]

In experimental models of nematodes (*Caenorhabditis elegans*) Bacopa improves stress tolerance and allows them to live longer.[429]

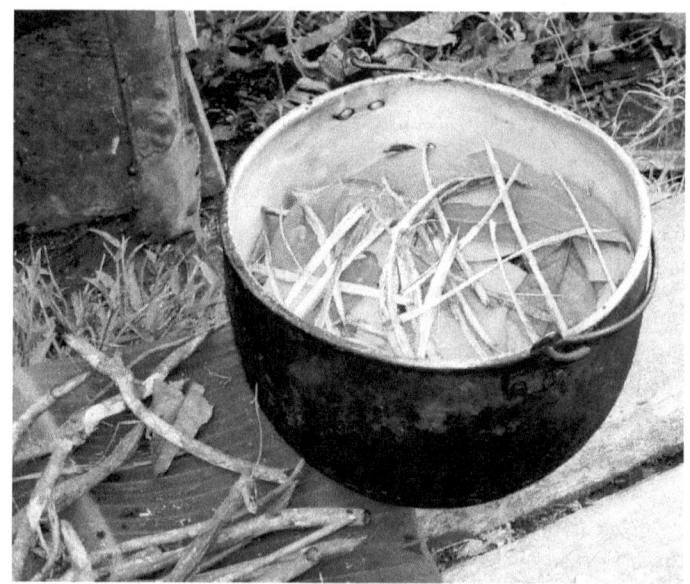

Ayahuasca and its main component, **Banisteria**, have peculiar psychoactive properties and very interesting pharmacological actions.

It may open horizons to improve treatment of Parkinson's disease, but its use is currently illegal and entirely contraindicated.

Ayahuasca and Banisteria

Monoamine oxidase inhibitors (MAOIs) occupy an important place in the treatment of Parkinson's but the first to be used was neither rasagiline (Azilect) nor selegiline (Eldepryl) but Banisteria, a vine from the Amazon. There was a media frenzy in 1929 when it was introduced as a "magical" treatment of post-encephalitic parkinsonism[484]; it later fell into oblivion, but recently has been resurrected and may offer new therapeutic horizons.[330]

In parts of Amazonia and the Andes ayahuasca (yagé) is considered to be a magical and sacred potion. It is used by the native people in their social, spiritual and healing rituals.

It is a hallucinogenic concoction of vines and roots from the Amazon rainforest: Banisteria (*Banisteria caapi*) whose active ingredient is banisterine (or harmala) and chacruna (*Psychotria viridis*) containing a tryptamine-derived alkaloid.[76, 77, 454, 466, 615] Ayahuasca has been used to relieve symptoms of Parkinson's disease and other neurodegenerative disorders. [163, 484, 586]

From the early twentieth century, its consumption forms part of certain tribal religious ceremonies in Brazil. In recent decades other groups ascribed to these rituals have been organized all over the world. However, consumption of these plants outside of these particular contexts in their countries of origin is punishable by law.[466]

FUNDAMENTALS

Ayahuasca means "vine of the spirits". For thousands of years, it was consumed by native American people to aid in making decisions, for healing purposes, or to resolve family or tribal conflicts. It is mixed with tobacco leaves (*Nicotiana tabacum* and *Nicotiana rustica*), *guanto* (*Brugmansia sanguinea*) and *guayusa* (*Ilex guayasa*) a species of holly, similar to *mate*, to counteract its bitter taste and to prevent its hangover-like effect.

Banisterine (*Nicotiana tabacum*)[330], also found in tobacco leaves, is similar to harmine, another alkaloid with MAOI actions that is found in the husk of the seeds of the Syrian Ruda or harmaga (*Peganum harmala*).

Ayahuasca has psychotherapeutic properties associated with its strong serotonergic activity. In recent years this concoction has been widespread among laymen and Western scientists, given its enormous potential in many fields. Ayahuasca has antidepressant and anxiolytic effects, and has been used for impulse control disorder, for withdrawal symptoms of toxic drugs, to improve REM sleep, and to explore the subconscious in psychiatry.[129, 163, 466]

PSYCHOACTIVE PROPERTIES

Ayahuasca is a psychoactive drug and its effects can be detected on electroencephalograms.[456] It produces perceptual, affective, cognitive and somatic alterations with feelings of pleasure and satisfaction.[455] Ayahuasca provokes a kind of reverie lasting 1-2 hours, that allows full awareness of the content of images and emotions. It is therefore advocated in psychotherapy to "open" the subconscious.

In a study conducted on 25 people monitored before ayahuasca intake and for 24 hours afterwards, it was found that the critical processing of experiences was reduced while internal concentration increased, thereby approaching situations of full self-consciousness.[529]

MOOD CHANGES

In an extensive review of 514 publications about ayahuasca, 21 studies selected for the validity of their criteria showed that the ayahuasca and its various components (harmine and harmaline) clearly improved anxiety and depression.[129]

In a different study, a composite beverage of ayahuasca (including banisterine and other plants) was administered to rats, and the monoamine rate was increased in the amygdala.[110] Another study with ayahuasca in female rats has shown that it has antidepressant effects and produces a greater serotonergic neuronal activation in brain areas.[430]

Also in rats it was found that ayahuasca administered for 30 days interferes with contextual association of emotional events related to the activation of the brain areas involved in these processes.[148]

CELL CULTURES

Reports about improvement of patients with Parkinson's disease taking ayahuasca led to trials about its effectiveness in cell cultures. Inhibition of MAO in the striatum of rats was found, as well as an increase in dopamine release.[496]

MECHANISM OF ACTION

The main components of ayahuasca are concentrated in its dry, thick branches, and have been identified by HPLC (high performance liquid chromatography). Some components act as inhibitors of MAO-A and MAO-B (harmine, harmaline and tetra-hydro-harmine) and others enhance its powerful antioxidant capacity (pro-anthocyanidins, epicatechin and pro-cyanidin) .[483, 586] It is deduced that Banisteria can be useful for treating Parkinson's disease and other neurodege-nerative disorders. [483]

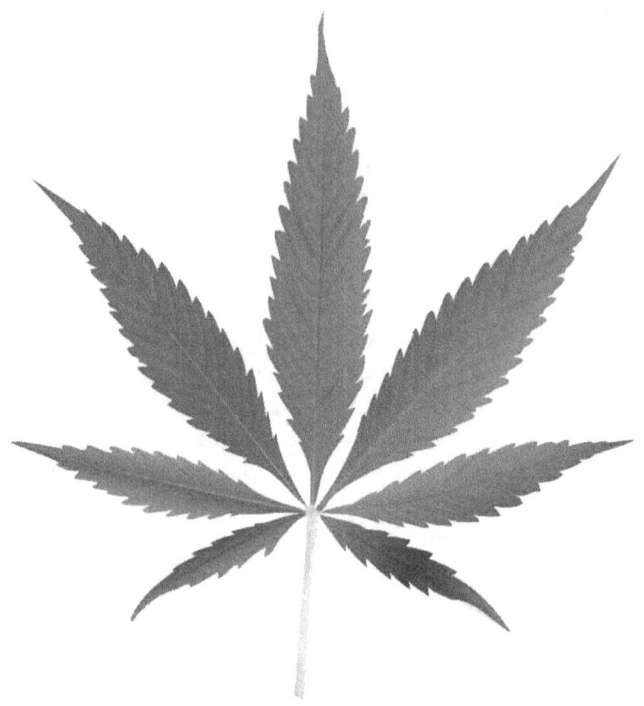

Cannabis (*Cannabis sativa*) contains substances that improve patients with abnormal movements. It has proven useful in treating tremor from multiple sclerosis, tics and dystonia; the results are less clear in hypokinesias and stiffness.

There are concerns regarding the potential for addiction, and the psychological or memory-related problems that may be induced by Cannabis.

Cannabis and Marijuana

Cannabis and its derivatives act on the dopaminergic system, have an antioxidant effect and prevent glutamate release in the striatum.[172] It is therefore suggested that it could slow the progression of Parkinson's disease and improve the quality of life of patients.[85]

Cannabis (*Cannabis sativa*) is a plant used to produce textiles and some varieties are rich in psychoactive substances (cannabinoids). Marijuana is a mixture of leaves, stems and flowers to be chewed or smoked; its main ingredient, tetrahydrocannabinol (THC), is concentrated in the center of the flowers. Hashish, an extract from the resin of the plant, has a concentration of THC eight times higher than marijuana.

CANNABIS AND PARKINSON'S

Cannabinoids modulate brain dopamine and motor activity in several ways: a decrease can improve tremor and dyskinesia, while at times it can cause hypokinesias.

These effects make cannabinoids (or selective antagonists) potentially useful for treatment of various symptoms of Parkinson's disease and other movement disorders. [84, 85, 387, 471, 500, 511]

FUNDAMENTALS

Marijuana does not cause physical addiction and coming off of it does not produce withdrawal symptoms, but it does cause psychological dependence. The effects appear in two phases: first, stimulation, dizziness and euphoria are experienced; later there is sedation and placid calmness. There are changes in mood and in perception of time and space, and the dimensions of the body seem altered. Other negative effects include: confusion, anxiety attacks, fear, helplessness, lack of inhibition or loss of self-control.

THE CANNABINOID SYSTEM IN THE BRAIN

Along with a dopaminergic or cholinergic system, our brain has a cannabinergic system, which works with cannabis-like substances (cannabinoids),[405, 457] and which influences movement, memory, pain and muscular contraction.[139]

Cannabinoids modulate other neurotransmitters in the basal ganglia. They are GABA-ergic (inhibitory), modify dopamine absorption[90] and inhibit glutamate[387] (and so are neuroprotectors).[336] In the same way that the body produces its own "morphine" (endorphins), it also has "endocannabioids" (brain chemicals with a marijuana-like effect)[139, 414] such as anandamide, which in Sanskrit means "inner happiness", a testament to the sense of wellbeing it produces.[591]

Tetra-hydro-cannabinol from marijuana activates the central and peripheral cannabinoid receptors and the brain's dopamine receptors (which, in the limbic system, launch "reward" responses). Cannabinoids, whether endogenous or exogenous, activate the mesolimbic dopamine system.[18]

THC causes changes in cognition, memory and perception,[147] promotes relaxation and produces a sense of wellbeing[403]; it also modulates the centers of appetite and vomiting, has an analgesic effect,[457] modifies the immune and inflammatory responses and motor performance (generally it decreases motility but the effects can be biphasic).[90]

MARIJUANA IN PHARMACIES

The finding that our body produces its own cannabinoids opens up new therapeutic horizons. Cannabis and its derivatives are used in patients undergoing chemotherapy (to relieve nausea), and is prescribed for chronic pain,[457] immune disorders, migraines,[480] epilepsy and multiple sclerosis.[361]

One pharmaceutical available since 1985, Marinol, is a synthetic derivative of tetrahydrocannabinol used for nausea and anorexia in cancer patients. Since 2003, a derivation of marijuana has been dispensed in pharmacies in the Netherlands in the form of a mouth spray. It contains tetrahydrocannabinol and cannabidiol that passes into the bloodstream by way of the buccal mucosa (the lining of the mouth). Its trade name is Sativex and is now sold in Spain as well, although it is expensive and requires an official narcotics prescription. In several European countries, as well as Australia, Mexico, Colombia and Israel, Sativex has been used successfully to control tardive dystonia.[3]

Currently, instead of marijuana or cannabis we should be talk ing about cannabinergics that are expanding treatments in the field of pain, immunosuppression, sedation, neuroprotection[362] and movement disorders[125, 336, 432] including dystonia[3] and Parkinson's disease.[182]

REM SLEEP DISORDERS AND DISKINESIAS

Cannabidiol (the major component of cannabis without the psychotropic effect) improved behavior disorders associated with REM sleep in four patients.[84] Several studies show that cannabis derivatives were effective in the treatment of levodopa-induced dyskinesias, tics, tremor and certain types of dystonia.[3, 26, 85, 387] They also modulate emotional states and would be an innovative therapy against anxiety.[258, 360]

Marihuana and hashish improve levodopa-induced dyskinesias in rats.[509] These dyskinesias are due to hyperactivity of the lateral part of the *globus pallidus*; when taking marijuana (or a synthetic agonist such as nabilone) there are cannabinoid receptors that are stimulated, thereby increasing transmission of GABA (an inhibitor) and the unpleasant dyskinesias are slowed.[509]

Methanandamide, analogous to the anandamide with more rapid (10 minutes) and more durable (over three hours) effectiveness, could be used in Parkinson's patients.[471] It may be beneficial in controlling dyskinesias and choreiform movements secondary to chronic levodopa therapy.[60, 471]

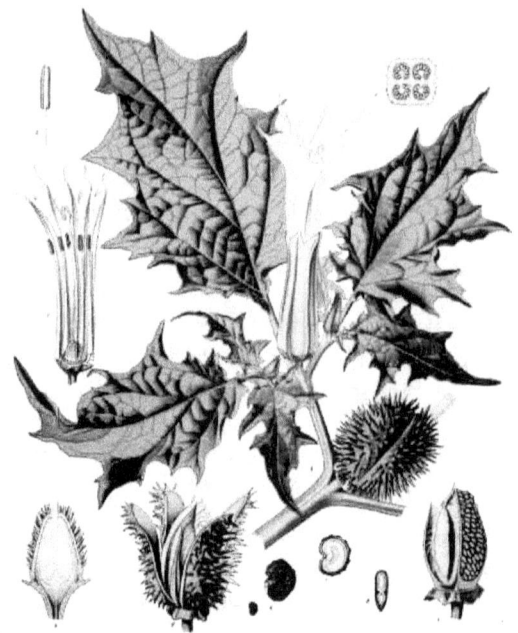

Other plants that influence symptoms of Parkinson's disease: Centella, Kampo herb, Galanthus, Ergot, Monk's pepper, Hypericum, Henbane, Jimson weed,...

Many are contraindicated and some of them may even worsen Parkinson's.

Others plants

There are many plants that have no direct effect on Parkinson's disease but can influence minor but frequent symptoms such as anxiety, depression, insomnia, constipation, sexual behavior (from loss of libido to hypersexuality), memory lapses, etc. I limit this section to the most commonly used plants and a few of historical interest.

CENTELLA

Centella or *gotu kola* (Centella *asiatica*) is an Indian plant used as a tonic and nerve stimulant that improves intelligence while it relaxes, and is considered to have a rejuvenating effect. Studies in rats confirm that it is a good antioxidant and improves cognition.[574]

Madecassoside is a major component of *gotu kola*; when given by gastric infusion to rats with MPTP-induced parkinsonism, it prevents nigrostriatal lesions, dopamine depletion and motor disorders.[604]

KAMPO HERB

The name Kampo is given to over sixteen types of Japanese herbs used in healing. A variety of Kampo (pronounced *kami-shoyo-san*) improves tremor of iatrogenic parkinsonism in two thirds of patients.[226] Given the diversity of species, dose, and effects, we do not recommend it.

GALANTHUS

In the *Odyssey*, Ulysses' companions are poisoned by the sorceress Circe with a plant that causes them to lose their memory and hallucinate, making them believe they have turned into pigs. That poison was most likely Jimson weed, a substance known to the Greeks and which contains anticholinergics that produce these symptoms.

Ulysses was not affected because previously the Gods had given him an antidote that was thought to be Galanthus, or snowdrop (*Galantus nivalis*).[433] This is a bulbous plant containing galantamine, a substance with the opposite effect of the Jimson weed because it is cholinergic, and is currently prescribed for dementia. Galanthus extract, or galantamine, may therefore be useful for Parkinson's patients with memory failure.[145, 183, 273, 472]

ERGOT

Several dopamine agonists such as bromocriptine (Parlodel), pergolide (Pharken) or cabergoline (Sogilen) are obtained from ergot (*Claviceps purpurea*), a fungus that parasitizes grain.

In the Middle Ages there were frequent intoxications from wheat, barley or rye colonized by ergot; it is chemically similar to lysergic acid (LSD) and produces hallucinations and behavioral disorders. In those times the psychoses were mistaken for witchcraft.[73]

There are tinctures containing ergot ergot which are highly toxic, and we advise against them absolutely. Formerly they were used to treat bleeding and headache and, in women, to facilitate labor and to treat menstrual disorders. Ergot (ergolines and ergopeptins) acts on the brain's dopamine pathways; therefore, ergot derivatives are still being sought after for treatment of Parkinson's, and would act in a fashion similar to the currently used dopamine agonists.

MONK'S PEPPER

The Latin adjective *'castus'* (chaste) refers to its property of calming sexual passion: *Vitex agnus castus* is the scientific name of "Monk's pepper", a substance that was used in monasteries to keep the libidinous impulses of their residents under control.

Monk's pepper is a bush, found along the Mediterranean coast and in Asia, bearing pink flowers and small berries. The plant has been used medically for two thousand years, particularly in women's disorders (menstrual problems, infertility, menopause). It is a hormone stabilizer that modulates progesterone and prolactin.[181, 231, 366, 522]

This herb is being investigated because its components are D2-dopaminergic agents (the most effective for motility) and inhibit prolactin.[231, 364]

HYPERICUM

Common St. John's wort (*Hypericum perforatum*) is a perennial plant widely used against depression but potentially dangerous. It contains hyperforin, a substance that inhibits the reuptake of serotonin, dopamine and noradrenaline.

It has demonstrated an antidepressant effect[76, 294, 334, 495] and, in theory, could boost the mood of Parkinson's patients. Its effectiveness as a nootropic and neuroprotective has been recently shown.[173] Moreover, when rats with rotenone-induced parkinsonism were treated with hypericum (enriched with hyperforin) mortality of dopaminergic neurons and motor symptoms were reduced.[173]

St. John's wort decreases the level of amitriptyline in the bloodstream, as well as that of warfarin, digoxin, theophylline and cyclosporine. It may cause problems when mixed with contraceptives (menorrhagia), antidiarrheals (delirium with loperamide) or antidepressants (serotonin syndrome with sertraline or paroxetine).[202, 227, 335] Because of the side effects and the risk of interactions, the use of hypericum is discouraged.[631]

HENBANE

Henbane (*Hyosciamus niger*) is a solanaceous plant containing several alkaloids (atropine, hyoscyamine and scopolamine) with anticholinergic properties, so it has been used to treat colic (it is spasmolytic) and various tremors, including in Parkinson's disease.

It should not be used because these substances are very dangerous and their proportions vary according to the variety of the plant and how it is marketed: usually as dry leaves and sometimes (still more dangerous) as seed extract.

JIMSON WEED

Jimson weed or Devil's snare (*Datura stramonium*) is another solanaceous, rapidly developing plant. The scent of the flowers contrasts with the nauseating odor of the leaves, which are a narcotic (as in the reference to the *Odyssey* above) and antispasmodic, as are the seeds.

They contain alkaloids such as atropine, hyoscyamine and scopolamine with an anticholinergic effect (similar to Artane or Akineton). Its effects are like those of Belladonna but more toxic: they disrupt memory, can cause confusion and even death in cases of misdosage. Strictly forbidden.

HERBS THAT PRODUCE PARKINSON'S

Some plants are neurotoxic and have been linked to the development of Parkinson's and other degenerative diseases.[76]

ALLELOPATHY

Plants need to protect their territory from surrounding species, and to that end they secrete toxins that attack their neighbors: this phenomenon is known as allelopathy. These toxins can affect humans as describe below.

Cyca and related plants (*Cycadaceae*) grow in tropical areas; it is shaped like a palm, although they are phylogenetically distant. In Guam and other Pacific islands, neurodegenerative diseases are found presenting as combined parkinsonism and motor neuron syndrome, and have been associated with the ingestion of the seeds of the cyca (*Cyca circinalis* and *Cyca rumphii*).[76] Other researchers think that the ingestion may be indirect, because the Chamorro Indians eat bats (cooked with coconut milk) which feed on cyca.[104, 621]

In the French Antilles, atypical parkinsonisms are frequently found associated with the consumption of various tropical fruits containing neurotoxic alkaloids.[72]

Patients should also avoid Kava-kava (*Piper methysticum*) which is used as a sedative. Kava interacts with benzodiazepines such as alprazolam (which may cause a semi-coma condition); it also increases 'off' (high symptomatic) periods in Parkinson's patients,[227] and induces buco-lingual dyskinesias and torticollis.[491]

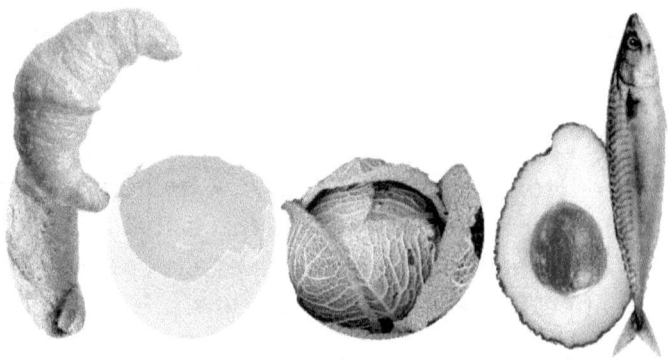

Food and **nutrient** are very similar terms, but nutrient is a more scientific one and has a more complex meaning.

There are non-energetic nutrients (vitamins and minerals) and *de facto* nutrients that also provide energy.

III. Nutrients

The promotion of nutrients that prevent aging and Parkinson's disease grows daily on the internet. A few of these 'miraculous' pro-ducts could help, but minimally: most of them neither heal nor hurt, and some may even be dangerous. The claims are based on assumptions, credible but unproven, that in Parkin-son's and other degenerative diseases involve some deficit (or excess) of substances necessary for cellular metabolism.[244]

Food and *nutrient* are very similar terms, but nutrient is a more scientific one and has a more complex meaning. There are non-energetic nutrients (vitamins and minerals) and *de facto* nutrients that also provide energy.

Vitamins and vitamin-like substances can affect Parkinson's. While no vitamin in isolation has proven effective to prevent or alleviate Parkinson's disease, some combinations of several of them may have some effect.

There are vitamin-like substances having similar actions to vitamins, with the difference that they are synthesized by the organism. Some of those that have been linked to Parkinson's disease are folic acid, coenzyme Q10 and flavonoids.

We also discuss here the energetic nutrients such as essential fatty acids, and nutrients from the ocean. In another book[178] I detail extensively other vitamins and nutrients, and here only describe ive major items in separate sections: multivitamins, folic acid, coenzyme Q10, omega 3, and polyphenols.

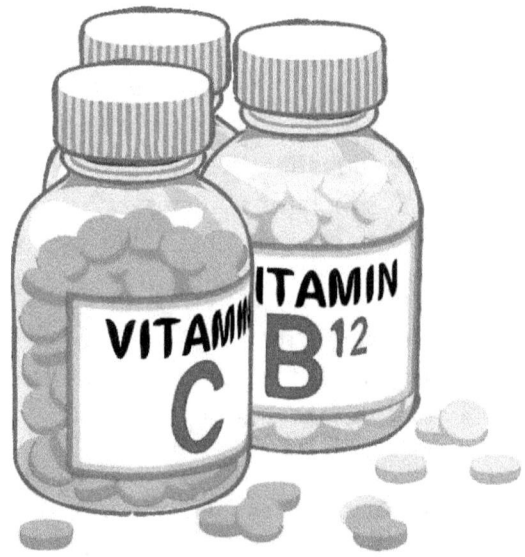

No **vitamin** or **nutrient** prevents Parkinson's disease, but some combinations of these may slow its evolution thanks to their antioxidant effects.

Patients in therapy with levodopa should take folic acid to reduce homocysteine in the blood. Some benefits have been observed in animals treated with Coenzyme Q10, flavonoids, resveratrol, essential fatty acids, and sea nutrients.

Multivitamins

Those who take multivitamins regularly have a lower risk of Parkinson's disease and, if they do succumb to it, symptoms appear some three years later.[322]

This study, published in the prestigious journal *Neurology*, involved 203 pairs of identical twins who share, of course, the same genes. In the cases where both siblings contracted Parkinson's disease, the individual taking vitamins regularly noticed symptoms later (3.2 years' delay on average).[322]

It is not possible to distinguish the effect of specific vitamins in isolation, but we do know the subjects were taking several, especially E, C, and A. The benefit may be thanks to antioxidants, which delay the onset of the disease, although they do not prevent it.[322]

Some governments (e.g. Israel) suggest giving all elderly people a standardized supplement with the minimum necessary doses of vitamins and minerals to prevent deficiencies.[130]

Folic acid

All patients treated with levodopa should take folic acid regularly to lower the homocysteine in their blood.

When homocysteine levels remain elevated the risk of contracting Parkinson's is increased[386, 610]; the same occurs for other neurodegenerative diseases, cardiovascular disorders and complications of pregnancy. [204]

Prescribing folic acid supplements for Parkinson's patients counteracts the perils of homocysteine. Taking this measure is both affordable and highly recommended.[351, 370, 385]

In adults, folic acid is neuroprotective, prevents physiological aging[345, 347, 349, 350] and decreases the risk of Parkinson's.[132, 351] Pregnant women, the elderly, and patients treated with levodopa should be given folic acid supplements.[350, 386]

FUNDAMENTALS

The name *folic* refers to the leaves of plants (*folium*, Latin for leaf), which are its main source; it is also contained abundantly in nuts.

Folic acid is essential to the processes of cell division and multiplication, both of which increase as a fetus develops, and so this supplement is prescribed preventively during pregnancy. Elderly people tend to have high levels of blood homocysteine and that can be reduced with folic acid supplements.[450]

Folic acid is necessary for the metabolism of nucleic acids and the formation of hemoglobin, and it performs another important function: the removal of homocysteine, a substance in blood that increases the risk of cardiovascular pathology, vascular dementia, and stroke,[347, 626] in addition to Parkinson's, depression, psychiatric disorders and cancer.[350, 351]

DANGERS OF HOMOCYSTEINE

People with Parkinson's disease have elevated levels of homocysteine in the blood,[70, 219, 386, 629] up to 30% above normal,[127] and homocysteine rises with increased age and the throughout the duration of the disease. The increase of homocysteine is accelerated when Parkinson's patients are depressed and when their levels of folic acid are low.[560]

The elevation of homocysteine observed in patients taking levodopa is lower when it is combined with entacapone (as in Stalevo)[569]; however lactic acid drops even further.[559] High homocysteine and low folic acid levels create an environment that favors neurodegeneration.

COGNITIVE IMPAIRMENT

Some researchers do not observe a relationship between homocysteine and cognitive impairment in Parkinson's patients,[70, 465] while others did: elevated homocysteine is frequently linked with increased risk of dementia.[48, 94, 338, 628]

Administering folic acid is a simple way to lower homocysteine and also prevent cardiovascular problems. The conclusion is clear: we should prescribe folic acid to every patient treated with levodopa.[127]

LEVODOPA-ASSOCIATED NEUROPATHY

Neuropathy is a complication of levodopa therapy that is usually moderate but relatively common. It is associated with increased homocysteine[83] and is more pronounced when it coincides with decreased levels of folate. [444]

ANIMAL MODELS OF PARKINSONISM

When mice with MPTP-induced parkinsonism are given folic acid they present fewer dopaminergic lesions.[132]

There is a genetic model of parkinsonism in fruit flies that is produced by modifying a Parkin allele, park(c00062). This mutation causes the fly to suffer developmental disorders, resulting in reduced size, higher mortality, disturbances in motility, and defects in mitochondrial respiration and cell metabolism. However, all these abnormalities are greatly decreased when folic acid supplements are given. It follows that by adding folate to the diet neurodegenerative diseases may be partially prevented.[536, 537]

Q-10 Coenzyme

Parkinson's patients have low levels of Coenzyme Q10 in the bloodstream[372] and some studies show improvements in those who take it for longer or shorter periods.[497, 611] Furthermore, those with the lowest initial levels of Q10 show the greatest improvements.[497] Animal models and cellular studies of Parkinson's show this enzyme, commonly known as "CoQ10", to be a neuroprotector.

CoQ10 is a fat-soluble vitamin-like compound found in almost every cell of the body (for that reason it is also known as ubiquinol, from *ubiquitous*). It intervenes in key processes for producing intracellular energy, and is also an antioxidant.

It is found in abundant quantities in animal organs, beef, sardines, mackerel and peanuts.[304]

Given that CoQ10 is essential for basic cell function, it is no surprise that it is prescribed for a many illnesses such as congestive heart failure, coronaropathy, and arterial hypertension.[282, 283, 304]

FUNDAMENTALS

CoQ10 is much more effective than vitamin E as an antioxidant and eradicator of free radicals. Q10 in the bloodstream decreases with age: after age 20, CoQ10 levels begin to decline, and so it is taken as a supplement to slow the effects of aging and to ward off neurode-generative diseases such as Parkinson's and others.[158, 159, 304, 515]

BENEFITS OF CoQ10 FOR PARKINSON'S PATIENTSs

Although exact average Q10 values are wide-ranging and difficult to define, Parkinson's patients are clearly deficient.[372] Coenzyme Q10 supplements slow the progression of Parkinson's disease. In one trial, daily doses of 300, 600, and 1200 mg per day were given. After 16 months, the study showed positive results: CoQ10 slowed functional decline with those taking a higher doses showing the greatest improvement. [516]

In a different study[497], 16 patients in the beginning stages of Parkinson's were given high doses (400, 800, 1200, and 2400 mg per day) for two weeks. The supplements were well tolerated and a significant clinical improvement was observed: their UPDRS (Unified Parkinson's Disease Rating Scale) went down and average of 27 to 37. The patients that had had the lowest Q10 levels in the blood initially showed the most improvement by far.[497]

In another recent long-term, random, double-blind, placebo-contolled study [611], 40 Parkinson's patients were divided into two groups. Group A patients were watched over a 48 week "wearing off" period, in which symptoms re-emerge before the next dose. The B group consisted of patients with early diagnosis but were not yet taking Levodopa, although they may have been taking other medications; this group was followed for 96 weeks. A portion of both groups took a placebo, and the rest took Q10 (reduced form, ubiquinole-19), 300 mg/day.

Over such a long period of time for the control, natural evolution of the disease would tend toward deterioration. At the end of the study, however, in group B (early diagnosis) those on the placebo had gotten worse, (UPDRS +5.1), as well as those who had taken the Q10 (USDRS +3.9). In group A (patients experiencing "wearing off") those taking the placebo deteriorated (UPDRS +2.9), while those who took the Q10 improved with a UPDRS decreased by 4 points (-4.2 +/- 8.2), after 48 weeks. This study clearly shows that CoQ1 produces long-term improvements in a particular type of patient with "wearing off". What is more, this treatment is safe and well tolerated.[611]

Other studies confirm the tolerability of Coenzyme Q10, but not its clinical effectiveness. Parkinson Study Group 2014 (208 collaborators) reported that CoQ10, while safe and well-tolerated, did not offer positive changes in symptoms.[420]

In a review of 4 selected randomized, double-blind, placebo-controlled studies with 452 patients with specific scientific criteria, treatment with Coenzyme Q10 (1200 mg/day for 16 months) was well-tolerated and resulted, using the UPDRS scale, in positive effects for daily activity, although this result is less conclusive, and more case studies are needed.[310]

CO Q10 IN ANIMAL MODELS

This treatment protects rats that have been parkinsonized using MPTP[157, 159, 495] as well as animal models for ALS.[341]

In mice, parkinsonism induced with sub-chronic infusion of MPTP produced a continual process of nigrostratial degeneration (loss of neurons and reduction of dopamine), which can be ceased by infusing drinking water with CoQ10 (such as Ubiso-Q10, a nanomicelle formulation with high bioavailability to the brain).[510]

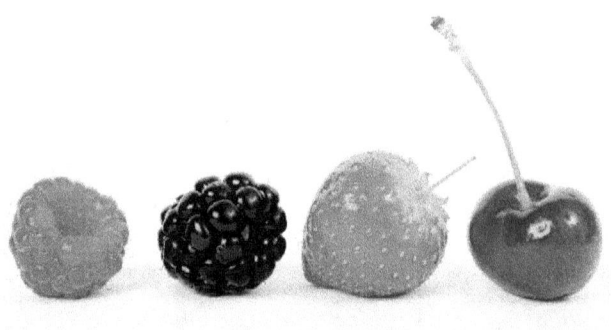

Flavonoids (polyphenols), antioxidant pigments found in plants and fruits, are very beneficial in treating Parkinson's and other neurodegenerative diseases. These anthocyanidins come in fruits ranging the color spectrum: blackberries, raspberries, strawberries, cherries, blueberries...

Naringenin is found in citrus fruits and is known to protect the substantia nigra in animals with toxin-induced parkinsonism.

Flavonoids

Flavonoids (a variety of polyphenols) are found in fruits and vegetables as well as in wine, tea, and chocolate. These compounds ferment in the human body, activated by bacteria that live in the digestive tract, creating metabolites that can be beneficial in Parkinson's and other neurodegenerative disorders. It works thanks to its antioxidant content and to other neuron-protecting mechanisms[225]: they act on the mitochondrial functions and on neuroinflammatory mechanisms, they limit deposition of protein aggregates and activate apoptosis.[236]

Speaking of green tea and chocolate, we should mention that they have many properties derived from their polyphenol content, more concretely, from their flavonoids. Other important sources of polyphenols are berries, black tea, beer, grapes (including wine), broccoli, pomogranates, walnuts, peanuts, olive oil, soy, *yerba mate*, and other fruits and vegetables. In fruits, the highest levels of polyphenols are generally found in the peel, so assimilation is best when fruit is eaten intact.

Only a few plants (and some algae) contain flavonoids, chemical substances that have more than one phenol group per molecule. They are really pigments responsible for the color in their flowers, to attract pollinators, and in their fruits, to attract animals that eat them and later disperse the seeds. In carnivorous plants these same colors attract the prey. Flavonoids also protect plants from intense ultraviolet radiation, and fend off herbivores with their unpleasant flavors.

FUNDAMENTALS

Flavus is Latin for yellow, but flavonoids take on other colors in plants: the buds are reddish, as are autumn leaves, and, depending on the soil, they can turn more bluish (alkaline soil) or violet (neutral soil).

There are over 600 major flavonoids (among over 9,000 known to date) found in fruits and vegetables, and most are healthy for humans. For the purposes of Parkinson's disease, we will highlight three: naringenin, nobiletin, and the anthocyanins.

ANTHOCYANIDINE

The anthocyanins are pigments found in fruits whose colors vary from red to blue or purple: blueberries, raspberries, blackberries, cherries, grapes, and plums.

An extract of blackberries rich in anthocyanins has proven be a neuroprotector in cell cultures and animal models of Parkinson's. Applied preventively in altered SH-SY5Y cells with 6-OHDA prevents lesions of dopaminergic neurons. In rats with subacutely MPTP-induced parkinsonism, the blackberry extract (alcohol 70%), applied as pretreatment, diminished hypokinesia and damage to the nigrotriatal neurons.[267]

In another trial using cellular models of Parkinson's, the neuroprotective ability of various fruit extracts rich in anthocyanins and proanthocyanidins, or other polyphenols, were compared. It was observed that extracts of blueberry, blackcurrants, blackberries, and grapeseeds protected cells from the effects of neurotoxins of retenone. It is deduced that anthocyanins can represent a new generation of bioactive drugs useful for Parkinson's symptoms or to treat Parkinson's[539, 236] and other neurodegenerative diseases.[236, 528]

NARINGENIN AND NOBILETIN

Naringenin, a flavanone from citrus (grapefruit) and some grape varieties, acts as a neuroprotector in animal models of Parkinson's, preventing lesions in rats by 6-OHDA,[266] and in cell cultures.[249, 298] Naringenin activates the production of neurotróphic factors and inhibits neuroinflammation, for which it one supposes that is a natural neuroprotective product of the nigrostratial domaminergic system.[298]

Nobiletin, a flavonoid found in mandarins, is neuroprotective in animal models of Parkinson's, preventing lesions induced by MPP+ (methyl phenyl pyridinium).[237] In rats with MPTP-induced parkinsonism, nobiletin improves motor disorders and cognitive deficit.[605]

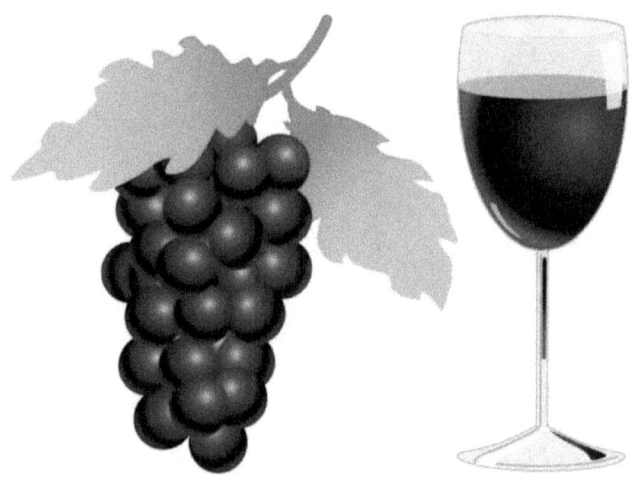

Resveratrol is found in red grape skin and red wine. It activates sirtuin, an enzyme that influences genes and prolongs life in laboratory animals.

It is an antioxidant and prevents the lesions to neurons in animals with toxin-induced parkinsonism. There is insufficient evidence of their effect on humans.

Resveratrol

There is an enzyme that prolongs life by the name of sirtuin. It is found in our cells and in those of plants and other animals, even bacteria and yeast.

By activating sirtuin with resveratrol (a polyphenol from red grapes and other berries) Dr. David Sinclair was able to prolong the life of yeast by 70%. That is the equivalent of prolonging our human life from 85 to 144 years! This is not mere talk from a medicine man at a state fair; the source was a publication in *Nature* by a Harvard scientist.[218]

Parkinson's, like other neurodegenerative diseases, is linked to longevity and the aging process, so resveratrol could fight it by activating sirtuin, which lengthens the life of cells. It also appears to be a panacea to combat Alzheimer's, Huntington's, etc.

For this reason Sinclair, a biologist, founded Sirtris Pharmaceuticals which focused on developing sirtuin activators to prolong life. The pharmaceutical company Glaxo paid $720 million to acquire what was presented to the press as a "modern-day fountain of youth". Rival laboratories put this claim in doubt.

Due to the low bioavailability of resveratrol, its pharmacological effects did not prove commercially viable, but its discovery led to the development of SIRT, another type of activator. A series of scientific debates led to the conclusion that the original findings were correct and that resveratrol and other synthetic compounds activate sirtuin 1. In 2014 both of these compounds (SRT1720 and SRT2014) were showed to prolong life and increase health in rats with a standard diet.[374]

FUNDAMENTALS

Resveratrol is a non-flavonoid polyphenol (phytoalexin) present in red grape skin, blueberries, raspberries, blackberries, and red wine. Sirtuin is an enzyme whose energy regulates longevity as demonstrated in yeast, larvae and fruit flies. Reseveratrol can activate sirtuin, which in turn can increase longevity and protect from neurodegenerative disorders such as Parkinson's, Alzheimer's, Huntington's, etc...[113, 220, 552]

ANIMAL MODELS

Administration of resveratrol (50 and 100 mg/day) for one or two weeks to mice who were later parkinsonized with MPTP intraperitonal prevented the depletion of striatal dopamine and decreased damage to nigrostriatal neurons.[50] Resvertatrol also protected rats with 6-OHDA-induced parkinsonism against these same lesions in dopaminergic neurons.[585]

Pretreatment with resveratrol in rats with MPTP-induced parkinsonism protects against lesions of the dopaminergic neurons of the substantia nigra and against dopamine depletion.[20] The same results were found in a model using mice with MPTP administered nasally. Mice that received resveratrol for 15 days (in nanoparticulates via the intraperitoneal route) were protected against neurochemical changes and behavioral alterations.[106]

CELL CULTURES

Resveratrol and oxi-resveratrol (from various berries) given as pre- and post-treatment in cell cultures of dopaminergic neurons (of neuroblastoma S-HSY5Y) act as neuroprotectors, by which we can extrapolate that they may have the same effect on Parkinson's.[89]

MECHANISM OF ACTION

Resveratrol acts by means of its antioxidant properties. Its anti-aging effects are due its activation of sirtuin, its anti-inflammatory action in the microglia, and its defense against lesions from the accumulation of alpha-synuclein.

The aging process is closely related the appearance of neurodegenerative disorders, especially Parkinson's and Alzheimer's. An ideal treatment would combine the effects of anti-aging and neuroprotection. Resveratrol is a good option due to its low toxicity and its antioxidant properties, and because it has demonstrated anti-aging effects in rats, yeasts, Caernorhabditis nematodes, and fruit flies, although the mechanisms have yet to be made clear. One hypothesis is that resveratrol activates Sirtuin 1 and modulates other proteins.[113, 220, 413]

Resveratrol activates sirtuin, proteins with epigenic action that modulates embryogenesis, neurogeneration, and other metabolic processes.[14, 15]

Furthermore, Sirtuin 1 is involved in the process of neuronal plasticity and the memory formation by epigenetic activation. This has been demonstrated in transgenetic mice that don't express the SIRT1 protein in brain tissue: the absence of sirtuin results in a decrease in neurons in the hippocampus (so important for memory) as demonstrated by serious errors on memory-based learning trials.[169]

Inflammatory microglia reactions have been observed in the substantia nigra of Parkinson's patients.[594] Resveratrol has neuroprotecive effects in animal Parkinson's models, specifically in rats inoculated with 6-OHDA, leading to a reduction of inflammatory reactions of the microglia.[243, 619]

In transgenic models using fruit flies (Drosophila) with parkinsonism induced by alpha-synuclein accumulation, locomotion disorders (progressive difficulty in jumping), loss of dopaminergic neurons of the substantia nigra are produced; when fed a botanical extract that includes grape (Vitis yinifrera) with resveratrol and other polyphenols, mobility (en males) is improved and longevity (in females) increases.[314]

APPLICATIONS FOR HUMANS

We wish to point out that experiments with resveratrol in animals or cell cultures are carried out under conditions and using doses very different from those for humans who consume the product. According to the present data, resveratrol cannot produce the same benefits in humans and is only indicated for use as a dietary supplement.

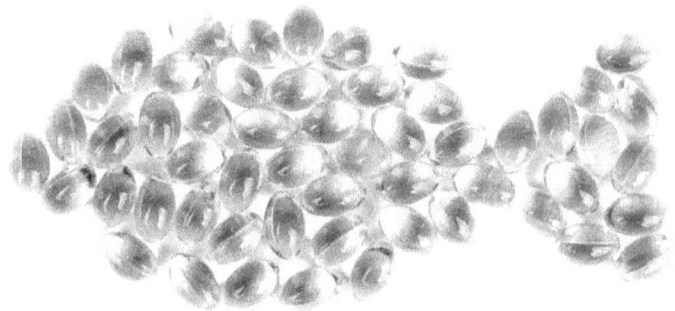

Essential fatty acids (such as Omega 3) are lipids that our bodies do not synthesize for themselves. They are found in oily fish, flax oil, and supplements.

The lack of these acids results in neuronal damage.

A diet rich in Omega-3 can delay the onset or progression of Parkinson's disease, Alzheimer's and other neurodegenerative disorders.

Essential Fatty Acids

Taking Omega-3 will not eliminate temblor or stiffness in a Parkinson's patient, but it could ameliorate symptoms or delay their onset in patients whose diets are rich in these essential fatty acids.[253]

If these lipids are missing in the diet, neurons are damaged and the brain becomes predisposed to Parkinson's, Alzheimer's, and many age-related problems. They are known as *essential* because the body cannot synthesize them and they must be ingested as food (salmon, sardines, tuna, flax seed, etc.) or in supplements.

A diet rich in Omega-3 fatty acids can delay the onset or the progression of these diseases.[614]

FUNDAMENTALS

Essential fatty acids are crucial to the monoamine neurotransmitter systems related to cognitive and motor processes.[422] They also modulate the chronic inflammatory responses activated by aging, which damage neurons and other cells and give way to neurodegenerative diseases. This is why they are so beneficial to older individuals, who should be encouraged to take them.[512, 557]

STUDIES IN HUMANS

Those who maintain a diet rich in essential fatty acids (Omega-3s, alpha-linolenic acid) are less likely to contract Parkinson's disease according to the meta-analysis of nine clinical studies.[253] Similarly, among farmers exposed to pesticides (paraquat and rotenona), those who ingested Omega-3s developed fewer cases of Parkinson's.[253]

Epidemiological studies and other research indicate that the ingestion of Omega-3 fatty acids and their polyunsaturated derivatives improves the immune system, prevents inflammation and cardiovascular disease,[35, 519,]

[545] and improves cerebral and peripheral nerve function. Low levels of Omega-3 have been observed in people with schizophrenia and some professionals propose treating them with dietary supplements.[246]

In a recent review of 21 studies which followed 4,438 cases over many years (from 2.1 to 21 years), an increase in fish consumption of one serving per week was associated with a lower risk of dementia and minor cognitive deterioration.[620]

ANIMAL MODELS

In rats with 6-OHDA-induced parkinsonism, striatal denervation and loss of dopaminergic neurons in the substantia nigra was observed. Three weeks later, a diet enriched with DHA (docosahexanoic acid) was administered for six weeks, and an increase in dopamine levels in the striatum was produced, by which it was deduced that DHA induces partial reparation.[103]

Young rats with diets low in linoleic and alpha-linolenic acids lose dopaminergic neurons in the midbrain and show oxidative stress lesions in the substantia nigra, even more so in the second generation.[74, 75, 422]

Even milk these days comes enriched with Omega-3 fatty acids. This means that it contains essential fatty acids (such as linoleic or alpha-linolenic) and their longer-chain derivatives or PUFA (polyunsaturated fatty acids) which are crucial to neuronal membrane function.

The most essential of these is alpha-linolenic acid, necessary for the formation of the more complex PUFA (arachidonic, eicosapentaeonic, and docosaehexonic acids).[519] The ability to synthesize PUFA decreases with age, especially in the presence of Parkinson's or Alzheimer's.

FLAX, PRIMROSE, AND EVENING PRIMROSE OILS

These are plants which contain valuable Omega-3 acids (and other similar ones such as Omega-6 and Omega-9), which are in such short supply in Parkinson's patients, and which are so hard to find in a normal diet. It is also important to pay attention to the proportions of each one.

In flax seed oil, obtained from flax seed, the major player is alpha-linolenic acid (Omega-3 group), and evening primrose is abundant in gamma-linolenic (Omega-6 family). Capsules of primrose oil, containing both Omega-3 and Omega-6 with oleic acid (Omega-9) are available for sale.

Diets including primrose oil are good for nerve conduction in rats with experimental diabetes.[199] In diabetics it improves lesions of the autonomic nervous system,[514] also damaged in Parkinson's patients, so they can also benefit from it. We need to wait and see how efficient it will prove to be.

NUTRITION FROM THE SEA

The oceans provide nutrients and biomedical substances that have novel applications. Commercial marine products of all types are sold, from algae concentrate to fish fats. Advertising can exaggerate the benefits, but at least these products are healthy. Some Omega-3 fatty acids are found in fish and other marine organisms.[519] It is abundant in oily fish, which contain over 5% fat by weight necessary for its high level of activity. "White" fish, on the other hand, is considered "sedentary" and is less nutritious despite being recommended in outdated diet plans.

The indigenous people of Alaska have elevated plasma concentrations of polyunsaturated Omega-3 fatty acids (up to 10 times above average), and levels vary by their geographic locations and according to the amount of fish and marine mammals they consume.[418]

There are marine fat concentrates (for example, Super-EPA) advertised as purified fish oil rich in Omega-3 fatty acids. They claim to be obesity-fighting fats that help lower cholesterol and triglyceride levels, repair tissue damage and protect against depression, Alzheimer's and Parkinson's.

N-3 polyunsaturated fatty acids of marine origin are neuroprotectors and provide cardiovascular benefits.[66, 67]

Finally, cod liver oil is good for pregnant women who want to have smarter children. This is not propaganda, but a prestigious study: cod liver oil contains long-chain Omega-3 fatty acids and the children of people who took it had an IQ significantly higher (measured at age four).[200]

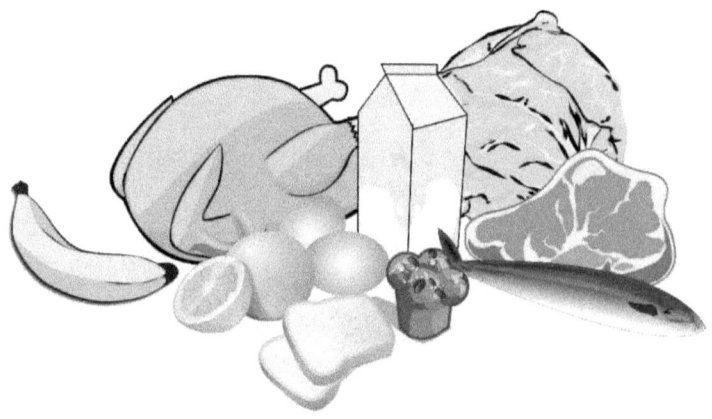

A Parkinson's patient should follow a balanced, natural, reduced-calorie **diet**, rich in carbohydrates, and put off protein consumption for night time, include lots of fiber and liquids, and eliminate animal fats.

In this chapter, we will discuss various diets: *ones that redistribute protein, are rich in carbohydrates, that adhere to vegetarian or Paleo guidelines, raw foods, fasting, etc.*

IV. The Nutritious Diet

Some people are fully lucid at age 90, while others suffer from "old brain syndrome" at 50. The difference depends on their genes, how they live, and what they eat.[348] While no food, vitamin, mineral or nutrient cures Parkinson's disease, a balanced, nutritious diet is very beneficial, delays aging, and decreases the risk of neurodegenerative diseases.[580, 583] It is also helpful if the diet is low in calories, rich in fiber, water and other liquids, and includes supplements and periods of fasting.

1. THE NUTRITIVE STATE OF PARKINSON'S PATIENTS

In the first stages of Parkinson's, there is weight gain due to the decrease in activity[40] or because some patients compensate for depression by eating. This is followed by progressive weight loss,[1] more so in women,[481] and even more pronounced when difficulty in chewing or lasting dyskinesias set in. Despite this, serious under-nutrition is rare.[1]

2. THE PROTEIN REDISTRIBUTION DIET

This is the most well-known. Amino acids compete with levodopa on two levels: during absorption in the intestines, and as they cross the blood-brain barrier.[193] In order to avoid this situation, Parkinson's patients who take levodopa should maintain a diet of protein redistribution: having protein at night and reducing the daytime intake to 10 grams. The benefits are evident in a week:[458] the efficacy of the levodopa is increased and motor fluctuations are decreased.

Done correctly, this plan does not affect the general nutritive state;[417] however, poorly managed cases can result in weight loss, a negative nitrogen balance,[581] a deficit of certain untrients and cognitive disturbances.[193]

In reality, it is not so much a question of when to take proteins as to lower their overall intake to less than 1 gram per kilo (.5 g per pound) of body weight per day.[78, 431] This is because the amount of amino acids circulating in the bloodstream at a given time have greater influence than the rate of their intestinal absorption.

3. CARBOHYDRATES VS. PROTEINS

We know that levodopa is poorly absorbed in the presence of proteins, and well absorbed in association with carbohydrates, but one must moderate the total amount of both substances. The best results are achieved by following the plan of *carbs-5, proteins-1*: in other words, to ingest five times as many carbohydrates as proteins (some suggest seven times more). This keeps the levels of amino acids and levodopa in the bloodstream stable, improves motor ability, and avoids fluctuations.[46]

Diets rich in carbohydrates and low in proteins increase longevity in animals. This will usually increase appetite and weight gain, resulting a complicated affair which we will simplify by resorting to the concept of the "nutritional geometry" framework. This is an analysis of relations between nutritional needs and how to meet them.[293]

4. THE FIBER-RICH DIET

A diet high in fiber will combat the frequent constipation that occurs with Parkinson's[262] and promote bowel movement.[607] Pharmacies and related stores offer various fiber supplements rich in cellulose and mucilage. These act as natural laxatives, forming bulk and absorbing liquids, but they should be taken under medical supervision.

Improving intestinal motility increases the absorption of levodopa and noticeably improves motor function.[31] We discussed this previously in the section on Plantago ovata.

5. THE VEGETARIAN DIET

Those who consume a lot of vegetables have a lower risk of contracting Parkinson's and other neurodegenerative diseases.[337, 356] Fruits and vegetables provide many antioxidants that are believed to delay the aging process and reduce the risk of, or the progression of, Parkinson's disease by neutralizing free radicals which damage neurons in the *substantia nigra*.

It appears that the protective action comes from the vegetables themselves because the administering antioxidants or vitamins alone does not produce significant effects.[311, 490]

It has not been clinically proven that fruits and vegetables benefit Parkinson's patients, but they are universally recommended.[53, 490] Those who subscribe to this diet complement their meals with juices that may even include vegetables. Tomatoes are particularly beneficial as they contain lycopene, a potent antioxidant.[442] Tomatoes increase dopamine levels in the striatum, act as a neuroprotector in mice, and could prevent Parkinson's in humans.[541] Feeding them freeze-dried tomato for four weeks is sufficient to protect them from MPTP-induced parkinsonism.[541]

6. THE MEDITERRANEAN DIET

The longer patients follow the Mediterranean diet, the lower their chances of developing Parkinson's disease, and the later it will appear in those who do contract it. This was found in a study of 250 Parkinson's patients over one year as compared to 198 control subjects.[16]

7. THE RAW DIET

There are those who promote a diet of 70% raw food.[11] Others are a bit extreme: according to their philosophy, in order to avoid not only Parkinson's, but most diseases, one must eat a strictly raw diet. Even vegetarians who boil their greens once a month will not pass muster; nothing that has been cooked may be consumed.

We will not go that far. Parkinson's patients, just like everybody else, should take in a good portion of raw food (fruits and vegetables)[201] and avoid overcooking those they prepare the stove.

8. THE Paleo DIET (AND Paleo LIVING)

Some predicate eating what cavemen ate before the dawn of agriculture. In Paleolithic times there were no chicken nuggets, macaroni and cheese, or bottled milk and, despite this, people were healthier. They also lived shorter lives, but this was a factor of their environment as well as their diet.

There are nutrients that have been with humans for 76,000 generations, such as meat, fish, eggs, forest fruits, greens and nuts. Others have accompanied us only 300 generations: processed foods such as refined sugar and vegetable oils, and there is a general consensus that these are not high quality nutrients.[424]

The optimal diet would be one for which we are genetically predisposed and, furthermore, we should return to living according to our bare necessities, as did our ancestors. We should redevelop habits that have been lost to modern life: eating when hungry and drinking when thirsty, exercise, and recovering our libido[404] (see the section "Paleo living" in the next chapter).

According to the Paleo diet, we need to eat carbohydrates, animal protein, and fats, as well as vegetables, fruits, nuts and edible algae. Fish should be on the menu seven times a week, preferable an oily variety, and shellfish. Dairy products are not essential, nor are legumes or grains, although they can be consumed on occasion.

The body needs carbohydrates, but not of the refined type. Farmed food should come from organic farms. One should eat only three times a day, and, of course, never snack.

As for drink, water is preferred, but only when one is thirsty. It is about changing habits and adopting a new (Paleo) lifestyle. Adults have no need for milk; humans are the only mammal that continue drinking it beyond childhood.

This cave dweller regimen has its detractors that consider it peculiar, and believe that eating patterns were no healthier during the Paleolithic, in part because people ate whatever they could: whether they brought down a mammoth or foraged for berries, dining was an opportunistic event.

9. LOW-CALORIE DIETING AND FASTING

Obese people between the ages of 45 and 65 have three times the chance of developing Parkinson's in future years.[3]

Limiting calories lengthens life, delays the aging process and prevents neurodegenerative disease.[165, 166] Fasting reduces oxidative stress in several organs.[62, 346, 575]

This the clear conclusion in experiments with mice and monkeys that suggest that a low-calorie diet decreases the incidence of Parkinson's in humans.[133, 346]

A hypocaloric diet protects the neurons because it increases antioxidant proteins, stabilizes intracellular calcium concentrations, and inhibits apoptosis. It also increases sirtuin, a class of beneficial proteins that are said to lengthen life.[166] Furthermore, the adult brain generates new neurons, which suggests that fasting increases neuroplasticity and self-reparation in the brain. It is interesting that most religions require some sort of alimentary restraint. Fasting causes extreme stress on the endocrine functions and the autonomic nervous system modifies itself accordingly.[544]

Parkinson's patients need to reduce their caloric intake, and some professionals recommend fasting, in other words, an extreme hypocaloric diet, several times a month.

10. DIET AND THE RISK OF PARKINSON'S

Consuming certain foods can influence the development of Parkinson's disease.[201] We can affirm the following, with a few discrepancies:

There exists a higher risk of Parkinson's among those who ate mushrooms during childhood,[578] or those who consume large quantities of animal fats,[21, 244, 311, 312, 356] dairy products (in males), sweets or foods with added sugar.[201, 490]

There exists a lower risk of Parkinson's in those who frequently eat ham, eggs, bread (the sandwich type or baguette), [144, 588] or potatoes.[201] Eating nuts and meat also protects against the disease,[588] especially those eaten raw or lightly cooked.[201]

11. MACROBIOTICS

The macrobiotic school of wholistic medicine originates in the far East, namely by George Osawa of Japan, and considers what we eat to be fundamental pilar of our health. The goal is to reach a balance between the body's *yin* and *yang*, while avoiding the intake of toxic substances; in this way a perfect balance is achieved, not only physically but also mentally and emotionally.

The macrobiotic regimen prefers foods of vegetable origin that are free of any chemical fertilizers, herbicides or pesticides, and that are not products of synthetic farming methods. Staple foods are legumes, marine algae, vegetable fats, soy and whole grains. One does not choose among these products, but rather combines them in proportion to the opposing but complementary "forces" that they possess. It is not necessary to subscribe the *yin-yang* philosophy in order to understand that health, for a Parkinson's patient or anyone else, improves when these natural foods are consumed in a balanced manner.

12. A DIET FOR THE PARKINSON'S PATIENT

In conclusion to this chapter, a Parkinson's patient should follow a balanced, natural, low-calorie diet rich in carbohydrates and avoiding animal fats. They should plan their protein intake for nighttime, and consume abundant liquids and fiber.

BALANCED: A balanced diet provides enough vitamins and minerals. It can include vitamin and mineral supplements, but in small quantities only. If there is concern about a lack of any nutrient, it is best to consume more of the foods known to contain it.

LOW IN CALORIES: An excess of calories worsens health, decreases longevity and quality of life, and can lead to neurodegenerative disease.

NATURAL: Avoid highly processed foods and, whenever possible, choose organic food grown without chemical fertilizers, insecticides or pesticides, packed without chemical preservatives.

VEGETABLES AND FIBER. A high intake of fiber, fruits, and vegetables (preferably raw) is recommended. It is a good idea to develop a taste for tomatoes and nuts.

DOWN WITH ANIMAL FAT. Avoid it.

UP WITH CARBS. The diet should include five times more carbohydrates than proteins.

PROTEIN AND LEVODOPA. Proteins (meat, fish, eggs, etc.) decrease the absorption of levodopa, especially when taken together. The medications should be taken 30 - 40 minutes before eating. Proteins, while necessary, should be eaten in reduced quantities during the day, preferably having them for dinner or later.

BOWEL MOVEMENT AND CONSTIPATION. Problems with emptying the stomach, constipation, and slow bowel move-ment interferes quite a bit with the absorption of medi-cations. Medications are not absorbed in the stomach, and if they remain there too long, they will deteriorate before passing to the intestines, where they would be absorbed. Slow movement of the bowel is also problematic. The solution is a diet rich in fiber, with abundant liquids and, if necessary, a supplement of *Plantago ovata* or some other bowel move-ment support.

13. THE FUTURE: NUTRIGENOMICS AND NUTRIGENETICS

We have moved beyond the concept of the nutritional diet, of foods that are beneficial or harmful. Today we talk about nutritional genomics: how nutrients modify gene function in general and for each person individually.

Nutrigenomics studies the exchange between nutrients and the genome, in other words, the effect of bioactive components of our diet on gene expression, and how these changes influence the cellular metabolism.

Nutrigenetics focuses on individual genetic variations. Over 99% of our genetic structure is the same for all humans, but a small percentage determines individual characteristics for each of us. Because of this relatively small variation, nutrients that are beneficial for some can be harmful for others. This fact is evident in some diseases: people with metabolic problems should avoid foods that are good for most others.

This idea brings us to the concept of the personalized diet, which would allow our cells to be optimally healthy and resistant to Parkinson's disease and other neurodegenerative disorders.[582] For now, however, we need to be satisfied with nutrients that, according to epidemiological studies, are helpful for the majority.

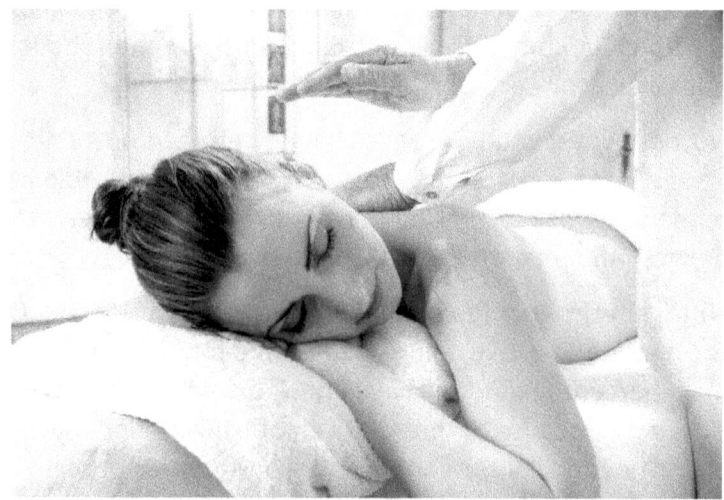

Just as there are gastronomic diets, there are also *sensory diets* that require adequate sensorial stimuli.

Therapeutic massage is highly recommended for Parkinson's patients for muscle stiffness and brady-kinesia, and to avoid muscle contraction, maintain mobility, relieve fatigue from temblors, reduce stress, facilitate sleep, and provide overall well-being.

V.The Sensory diet

It is enough to merely touch a Parkinson's patient to alleviate or even "melt" a frozen muscle. The body should be touched, caressed and massaged, which is good for all of us, but proves particularly valuable to Parkinson's patients.[178]

Along with the nutritional diet, there is a sensory diet that requires certain sensory stimuli. While the stomach feeds on potatoes or meat, the nervous system is fed with sensory stimuli: the brain consumes color, odors and flavors. Without these, it atrophies, withers, and declines.

Parkinson's patients are infrequently touched and they rarely "rub elbows" with others (neither physically nor mentally). Many have their mental functions intact, but lose control of their bodies: they find themselves consciously in possession of failing flesh and bones, aware that their limbs need attention and care.

Our bodies belong to us, and should be enjoyed, touched, and stimulated. Tactile experience contributes to the sensory diet through massage, caressing, and other types of touch. Nerve-based nutrition is rounded out through olfactory, gustative, visual and auditory sensory input, all of which can be incorporated into a massage experience. Massage reestablishes the lines of communication to our bodies and our senses.[277]

MASSAGE AND CARESSING

The word *massage* comes from the Greek *masein* and from the Latin *massa* (to knead). It describes a manner of contact or touch that manipulates the skin and muscles against the bones with a kneading type of action,[69] and is most effective with the use of essential oils. It is a method for motor-sensory training: it awakens a flow of ancient sensory information which combines with the feelings newly generated by the experience. The wellness provided by massage is due to the endorphins that are freed in the process.[252] We are born to touch and be touched, and studies confirm what we can guess by intuition: touch and massage are the building blocks of a healthy body and mind.[277]

Physical contact has endocrinological effects and plays a vital role in cerebral and physical development, as has been demonstrated in children and animals.[358, 359] Laboratory rats which are touched and petted from an early age respond better to stress and experience delayed aging. The opposite also occurs: baby rats that are denied tactile contact lose neurons in the hippocampus over time and suffer from spacial memory loss quite early on.[358, 359]

THERAPEUTIC MASSAGE

Therapeutic massage consists of skilled contact meant to reduce injury-related pain, illness, or stress. In 1800 the Swedish researcher Peter LIng developed a scientific system for therapeutic massage by organizing basic maneuvers and techniques of traditional massage in line with the principles of the anatomy and physiology of the period.

During the polio epidemic (1920 - 1950), physiotherapists used massage frequently[260] although this method was later partially abandoned when machines were employed for exercise and rehabilitation. Today, massage has reemerged as the fastest growing complementary therapy,[69] the most commonly one used for Parkinson's patients (along with aromatherapy)[153] and, for the benefits received, is more affordable than acupuncture or chiropractics.[96]

Massage has mechanical, chemical, psychological, and reflexive effects, and its physiological fundamentals have been known for thirty years. It supports circulation in the bloodstream and the lymphatic system, decreases inflammation of the limbs, changes the temperature and metabolic processes of the skin, relaxes and revives fatigued muscles, increases articular mobility, and improves pulmonary, neuromuscular and autonomic functions.[146]

TYPES OF MASSAGE

The most common variety is Swedish massage in which essential oils are applied with the hands which glide over the skin exerting light pressure and delivering small taps. Deep tissue therapies such as neuromuscular, Rolfing, and trigger point therapy can be somewhat more uncomfortable, but produce effective results in some types of chronic pain.

Shiatsu is a type of massage originating in Japan which applies pressure with the fingers to different parts of the body (pressure point massage). It is effective for dysmenorrhea (menstrual cramps)[551] and postpartum nausea,[371] and boosts healthy sleeping and general quality of life in patients with chronic problems.[92, 563, 564]

Asian massage is understood to act on the corporal meridians and to normalize energy flow. Whether or not one believes the theoretical fundamentals, they prove to be useful in practice.

MASSAGE AS A GENERAL HEALTH PRACTICE

Massage has been institutionalized in some hospitals. Studies have shown that it improve relaxation (98%), a general feeling of well-being (93%), and mood (88%), promotes mobility and energy, and allows for greater participation and faster rehabilitation..[525]

The skin is the primordial organ through which childhood experience is inculcated. Massage relaxes profoundly and reduces stress in older patients, making them feel more protected and cared for,[59, 155, 156] and can even control behavioral problems from dementia[59, 448, 461] and schizophrenia.[22] It also relieves fatigue[146, 206] and improves sleep.[69] The lack of tactile contact in infancy is related to violent behavior in adolescence and this behavior is improved with therapeutic massage;[124, 155] it is also effective for children with autism.[105]

Using essential oils in massage provides the added benefit of aromatherapy. This can help with postpartum discomfort[550] and with chronic conditions (such as multiple sclerosis),[216] ictus (stroke),[210] cancer[192, 524] and pruritis (itchiness) due to kidney disease.[460] Neck and shoulder massage can relieve tension in the head,[438] rubbing the muscles of the abdomen can help relieve constipation.[435]

THERAPEUTIC MASSAGE AND PARKINSON'S

Massage is highly recommended in Parkinson's[333] for mobility and prevention of muscle stiffness, and it is best to apply essential oils along with it. Massage improves bradykinesia and muscle contractions, relieves fatigue caused by temblors[69]; reduces stress, facilitates sleep, and produces a general sense of well-being. [126, 543]

A massage therapist will work the limbs with rhythmic pulsations, alternating compression and tapping. The effect is to support blood flow returning to the heart, and to curb hypertonia (spasticity). Intermittent taps are applied in the case of muscle spams, and, once they subside, slow, continuous massage; later friction massage is applied to the more injured areas with passive stretching.[69] In cases of severe stiffness and hypokinesiaS, myofascial massage is applied with friction to tense ligaments in order to soften the tissues. To address edema (swelling) due lack of mobility, a gentle massage is used to assist in lymphatic drainage.[69]

Many Parkinson's patients cannot tolerate deep tissue massage, so Swedish massage or other gentle variations, are recommended, as long as the patient is in a comfortable position (some cannot tolerate lying face-down) and the room temperature is comfortable, as thermal variation can is so unbearable for patients.[635]

Self-massage is another option. Parkinson's patients can and should massage themselves as much as possible using wooden rollers or massage balls.[633] Some use vibrating massage for stiffness, although this does not produce consistent results.

THE VIBRATING CHAIR (OR *CHAISE TRÉPIDANTE*)

A peculiar Parkinson's "treatment" brainstormed by the prestigious neurologist Jean-Martin Charcot has gotten a lot of attention.[175] Observing that Parkinson's patients improved after long trips by train, he designed a type of "shaking chair" (*chaise trépidante*) with a crank and a series of gears and levers. The patient would sit, an assistant would turn the crank, and the device would produce a strange type of rattle, similar to a train.

Years ago, a colleague of mine[381] commented that a Parkinson's patient of his, a farmer, had a trick: each morning, before taking his Sinemet, he would take a ride on his tractor, and feel relief. If one considers this novel approach in the context of Charcot's apparatus and the train effect, something that would seem almost comical becomes a foundation for treatment: the act of shaking the limbs, aside from loosening them, is a way of activating proprioceptive sensitivity. Stimulation through vibration constitutes a part of a "sensory diet" for the "nourishment" of those parts of the central nervous system implicated in movement.

INSTINCT AND EMOTION: Paleo LIVING

Another form of nourishing the primitive brain is to seek elementary emotions and situations in which our basic instincts come back into play. This conforms with Loren Cordain's position on the Paleo diet.

A large percentage of health problems in modern society can be attributed to patterns of physical and mental activity that are vastly different from those our genetic makeup has prepared us for. Our genome was forged in the ancestors who survived within an environment of natural selection, one that required a high level of motor activity and energy exertion in order for our ancestors to be successful and prosper. They had to forage for fruits, run, hunt, fight... A vigorous, outdoor, lifestyle that is now lost. This activity enhances the circuitry of primitive neurons, of the limbic system and its neighboring structures, that are affected from such and early stage in Parkinson's and other neurodegenerative diseases.

In practice, these patterns would be replicated, simulating the routine physical activity of our hunter-gatherer ancestors: we should eat when hungry and drink when thirsty, exercise, and regain our libido.[404]

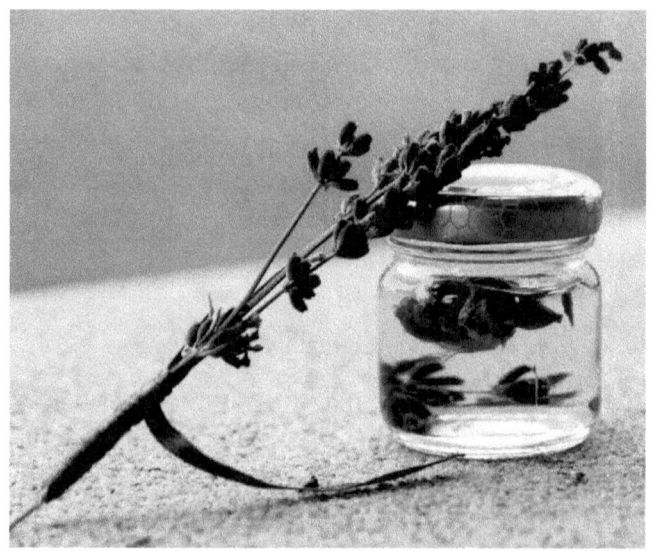

Aromatherapy produces emotional changes.

Applying essential oils or perfumes during massage encourages relaxation and produces a sense of general well-being that is very useful for Parkinson's patients.

VI. Aromatherapy

This forms part of the "sensory diet". Aromatherapy means treatment by means of aromas or perfumes that are applied either directly or with massage. It is assumed that this improves health and emotional well-being, restores physical balance and relieves various disorders. It is the preferred alternative therapy among Parkinson's patients.[153]

Babies recognize their mothers through scent, certain odors unpack ancient memories, there are perfumes that incite feelings of love, we shun strong odors. The nostrils are the shortest and fastest route to the brain.[33, 137, 195, 443] The olfactory nerve is not really a nerve but and extension of the brain that leads directly to the olfactory bulb and the limbic system (areas affecting emotion and memory).

This is why Proust (in his novel *In Search of Lost Time*)[436] by smelling and tasting his famous muffin as an adult, intensely relives childhood scenes thought to be forgotten. Science has confirmed what this French novelist knew by intuition: certain odors bring back memories that were created in their presence.[523]

GENERAL THOUGHTS

Aromatic plants were used as cosmetics and medicines in ancient Egypt, Classic Greece and Rome, and in China, India, and all of Europe up to the end of the 19th century, when they began to be replaced by synthetic pharmaceuticals. The term aromatherapy is used up to 1930, in which the French chemist René-Maurice Gattefossé studied essential oils.

Aromatherapy can be used to treat skin problems such as wounds and burns, respiratory disorders such as colds, cough and sinusitis, muscle pain, arthritis, rheumatism, headaches and stress-related symptoms like insomnia, anxiety, and depression. It is currently the fastest-growing complementary therapy. It is used in homes as well as private clinics and some nurses apply aroma as an analgesic and calming agent.[65, 388]

ESSENTIAL OILS

Essential oils are aromatic substances extracted from plants, usually with pleasant odors that have beneficial psychological and physical effects on the body. They are extracted from flowers, fruits, leaves, roots, seeds or bark. Lavender extract, for example, comes from the flower, pachouli oil from leaves, orange oil from the fruit. They are all highly concentrated and should be natural and pure.(BUCKLE 2000).

AROMATHERAPY, THE BRAIN, AND BEHAVIOR

We can distinguish up to 10,000 different odors and many affect us, without our knowing it, by acting on the brain. Specifically, they act on the amygdala, the hippocampus, and other areas of the limbic system related to mood, emotions, memory and learning.

Aromas have been shown to produce emotional changes and modify behavior in mammals.[264, 462] Chamomile has a calming effect and improves mood.[462] In some banks in Japan lavender and rosemary are dispersed near the customers to relax them while they wait, while the stimulating fragrances of eucalyptus and lemon are pumped into the other side of the counter to keep the tellers alert.[56] Lavender scent, however, provokes mathematical errors.[316]

Aromatherapy favors deep relaxation, alters pain perception and produces changes detectable on an electromyogram (EMG), an electroencephalogram (EEG), and in cardiac rhythm.[37, 272] Massage with lavender acts as an analgesic and its sedative effects are comparable with those of Valium.[64] It is used to help control patients with dementia and major behavioral disorders.[59]

There are certain odors that improve mental function or that have neuroprotective effects. Spanish sage (*Salvia lavandulifolia*) improves memory because it contains essential oils with monoterpenoids that inhibit acetylcholinesterase,[425] that is to say, it is the same mechanism that pharmaceutical companies produce for Alzheimer's and other neurodegenerative disorders.

AROMATHERAPY FOR PARKINSON'S

Pain and stiffness due to Parkinson's may be lessened by applying locally a compress containing the essential oils of ginger (*Zingiber officinale*) or common juniper (*Juniperus* communis) which supports circulation and relaxes the muscles. Marjoram is another muscle relaxant and is recommended specifically for Parkinson's patients with nocturnal muscle cramps.

One drop of chamomile or roman chamomile (*Anthemis nobilis*) oil rubbed into the solar plexus relieves mental or physical tension. Vaporizors with lavandar (*Lavandula vera officinalis*) are used for stress, or with rosemary (*Rosmarinus officinalis*) for fatigue and musucle pain, and, in the bedroom, chamomile or roman chamomile (*Chamaemelum nobile, Anthemis nobilis*) essence acts as an antidepressant and sedative (ROBERTS 1992), facilitating sleep.

In general, menthol and eucalyptus are used as stimulants. Bitter orange is a sedative, bergamot orange has antidepressive effects, and geranium promotes mind-body equilibrium. In the case of a particularly anxious state, a relaxing bath is recommended with a combination of lavender, geranium, and bergamot orange in sweet almond oil. To promote sleep, the bath would contain essential oils of roman chamomile and geranium[56]

A lavender bath produces a pleasant sense of well-being and dispels negative thoughts, angry feelings and frustration.[383]

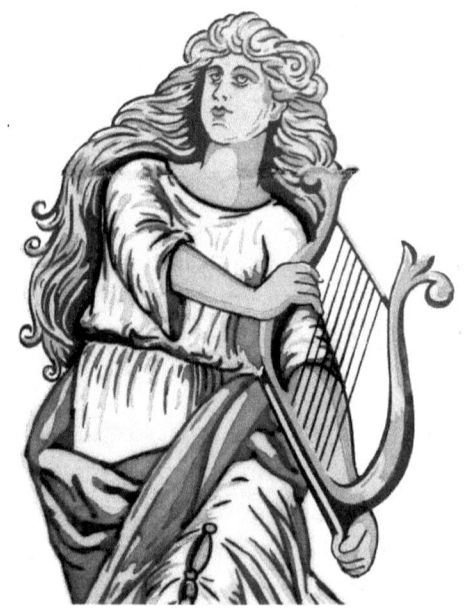

Music and dance can rewire damaged cerebral pathways.

In Parkinson's patients these activities can relieve symptoms and improve function and the functional capacity of the brain, providing the recipients with a needed kinetic melody, as it were.

VII. Music and dance

"Without music, life would be a mistake" affirms by Nietzsche. Music modifies mood, controls behavior, supports motor activity and contributes to the well-being of humans.

From antiquity, traditional medicine has included music in treatments. One of the earliest known examples of this is when David plays the harp to cure Samuel *Samuel 1, 16:23*). The Arabs developed a specific musical system to treat many illnesses from dementia to syphilis.

Music therapy is a recognized science.[339, 340] It has been shown to improve motor function, affect, and behavior, and music-based treatments are recommended as part of a rehabilitation program for Parkinson's patients.[410, 411]

MUSIC AND PHYSIOLOGICAL CHANGE

Music affects human physiology: it produces changes in respiration, cardiac rhythm and blood pressure; it lowers cortisol levels (which rise with stress), and it increases endorphins, the natural "feel-good" hormones.

The brain, especially the motor functions, are very sensitive to music and any other rhythm, and treatment can take advantage of this in rehabilitation for movement disorders.[556]

Not every type of music has the same influence on the brain. Classical music improves cognition,[80] possibly due to its rhythmic structure, and it is said that listening to Mozart can raise IQ test scores.

CLINICAL EFFECTIVENESS

Music is capable of rewiring damaged cerebral pathways making it very useful in neurological disorders. It has been shown that music can relieve symptoms and can improve gait and global functional ability in Parkinson's patients. Music therapy is used to treat stroke, cranial trauma, and dementia. It also relieves depression and anxiety and has analgesic affects.[274, 391]

Music is well-tolerated, does not cost money, is familiar and enjoyable to all, and has no collateral effects. However, there are precautions to observe: some people become agitated by music, others do not respond, and rapid beats are not recommended if serious heart problems are present. Not all music is good for everybody. Of course, the patient must like the choice of music.

MUSIC THERAPY AND PARKINSON'S

In Parkinson's, music acts as a stimulant to obtain motor and emotional responses by combining it with movement to activate different sensory pathways. Musical rhythm can synchronize muscular movements and regulate motor ability, making them more efficient.[410, 411, 617]

Music therapy (choral singing, voice exercises, free and rhythmic body movements, active music with group improvisation) is very beneficial for Parkinson's patients. It produces greater general motor performance, with benefits observed specifically for hypkinesias and bradykinesia. There is also an unmistakable emotional benefit, along with a significant increase in daily activity level and quality of life.[410, 411]

DANCE

Many Parkinson's patients who are barely able to walk can dance marvelously. Parkinson's patients can dance better than they can walk, and they must take advantage of this.

One can use common sense to tell the difference between a Parkinson's patient who does not exercise, stays home, does not socialize, and is lonely, compared to one who has a group of friends as an incentive to go out and dance. Whether if only for physical, psychological or social rehabilitation, dance is a tonic.

Ballroom dancing improves health in general in various ways: muscle exercise, ambulatory motion and amusement. It not only increases muscle mass in the limbs but it also improves balance by activating proprioceptive pathways and coordination; this has been observed specifically in computer assisted balance platforms.[286]

THE MELODY OF MOVEMENT

Parkinson's patients do not experience paralysis, rather their movements become slower and more infrequent. They struggle to coordinate and carry out the successive steps of each motion, to execute the "program" or "rhythm" of each gesture.

Their actions are not only slow and infrequent, but appear automatized, affected, robot-like. These patients lack what we call, and for good reason, the kinetic "melody" of movement, the tune or rhythm we move to.

It has been long known that Parkinson's patients learn "tricks" for walking when they freeze up: they mark each step as they go, using points of reference such as a cane or lines on the pavement, they take advantage of music that may be playing (an upbeat military march is best) or use other strategies. It is almost as if Parkinson's patients borrowed the rhythmic ability they lack from the surrounding environment. The benefit is greater for external auditory rhythms.[308, 535]

That is what music and dance does for these patients: it provides them with a beat, the "melodic" foundation of the musical program that their brains lack. Parkinson's patients improve quite a bit with dancing, but it is important to monitor the heart and to be very careful to avoid falling.

One interesting thing: the tango gets a lot of praise for its effectiveness in improving Parkinson's symptoms.[315, 459] Some suggest that the tango can improve balance and functional mobility, even modest benefits for cognition and fatigue are described.[459]

CHOOSING THE RIGHT DANCE FOR THE PATIENT

Along with music therapy, dancing is accompanied by or is alternated with exercises with rhythmic and synergistic patterns (for hypokinesia). Also useful are dances that stimulate emotionally (for temblor) and "free" dance which combines exercises for fluidity (to address stiffness).

Biodanza (literally, *the dance of life*) combines various modalities of dance associated with other rhythmic and therapeutic exercises. It can focus on particular symptoms, what is more important to the patient, or what he or she wants to address specifically.

In patients who struggle to start moving, slow, expressive dancing is used. If the issue involves complex motor sequences, abrupt changes in tempo are preferable (for instance, a samba beat is changed to a jazz or tango rhythm), and to address language disorders, dancing is combined with soft singing within the patient's range of ability.

For patients who are inhibited expressively, the choice is a dance that is creative and rich in original movements. For people who are shy or suffer from low self-esteem, the program would include dances that require frequent close contact with others and dances with specific, deliberate step patterns. Dancing works for everybody and can be personalized for the needs of each patient.

SONG

Marked improvements have been described in Parkinson's patients who join choral groups.[290] There are specific protocols for them with musical voice therapies that include singing and vocalization exercises.

In patients with language problems, singing helps make their speech easier to understand, and increases intensity, basal frequency and variations in pitch.[196]

If the main problem is hypophonia (quiet voice) an effective method of treatment, known as the Lee Silverman system, raises the volume of the voice.

PET scans and studies of regional cerebral flow shows that, when they attempt to speak, the brains of Parkinsons's patients are activated in the premotor and motor areas, or those associated with voluntary actions, and that after following this treatment the active areas during speech are reorganized to rely more on the autonomic pathways (the basal ganglia, the anterior insular cortex), as occurs in healthy people..[291]

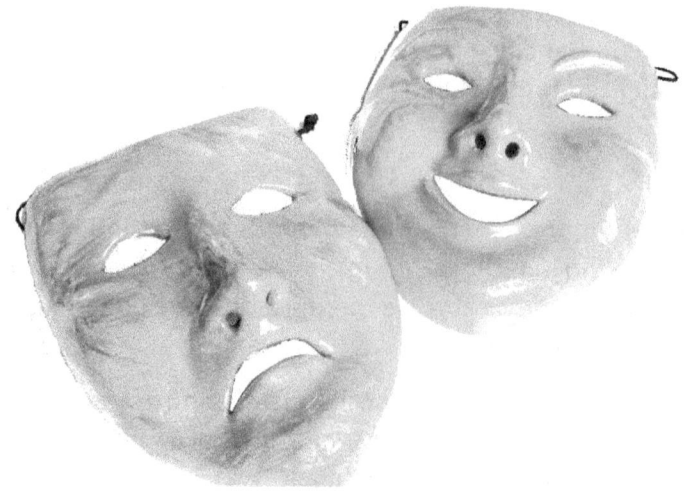

Parkinson's patients have poor strategies for dealing with stress and this increases their symptoms and aids progression of the disease.

They need an **emotional approach**, a way of channelling stress and enjoying life, to embrace a self-indulgent attitude. They should avoid others who are unhappy and dispel negative situations and thoughts.

VIII. Emotional hygiene

In school children are taught math and geography but not how to manage their emotions or cope with their feelings. This is certainly a life skill of the highest priority: to learn to regulate one's joys and conflicts, to maintain affective hygiene, to build a personality over time as if constructing a building, brick by brick, one characteristic at a time.

Parkinson's patients should be aware of the weaknesses in their personalities, their emotional economy, as it were, how they react to stress. This is a natural method of self-help, although it is most worthwhile if done with the guidance of a professional. A psychotherapist can teach us how to modify our behavior or how to manage emotions the same way we might learn a new language or computer skills. Psychotherapy improves symptoms of Parkinson's disease. Little by little, patients form a new attitude towards themselves and their environments, they alter their view of themselves and internalize the new vision. They begin to approach life from a new, more flexible and more enlightened angle.

It is said that Parkinson's patients have a special (non-dopaminergic) personality: they overreact to stress, possess rigid morals and poor emotional hygiene, they are prone to self-sacrifice, cannot enjoy life, and tend to become overwhelmed by their social and family relations. It would be helpful to try to turn some of these traits on their heads. Building tolerance and flexibility and practicing self-indulgence benefits Parkinson's patients.

Let us analyze five topics deeply engrained in psycho-therapy: personality, stress, self-indulgence, social and family support, and managing emotions.

1. DOPAMINE AND PERSONALITY

We do not wish to assert that tobacco protects against Parkinson's, but smokers' brains do in fact contain more dopamine, and this influences their personalities. It makes them more likely to smoke, but also to drink alcohol or coffee excessively, or to latch onto any addiction including thrill and adventure seeking.[592]

The opposite is also true: young people pre-disposed to Parkinson's possess a special personality characterized by a self-limiting attitude[242] towards tobacco, alcohol, and any other substance suggestive of drugs, danger or novelty. A prominent personality trait in patients is to avoid problems; they avoid danger to an unreasonable degree (typical depressive behavior)[257] miss opportunities for adventure, and show little or no interest in anything new.[369]

2. LEARNING TO MANAGE STRESS

Stress kills neurons and exacerbates or provokes the onset of Parkinson's disease. Chronic stress does even more damage, and how it is internalized is also a factor.

We all have bad things happen to us, that is life. But what affects us more than the incidents is how we "digest" them, in other words, how each individual reacts to adversity.[167]

Parkinson's patients have poor strategies for dealing with stress,[162] and they tend to perceive more intensely. They internalize more negative feelings when faced with life's circumstances. Anxiety is defined as a disproportionate reaction to stress. Stress or anxiety can intensify a freezing, or *off* episode.[342, 349, 476]

Patients must learn to respond to conflict with relaxation techniques, and use emotional education programs to lift their self-esteem and to free them from anxiety.

3. *SAVOIR-VIVRE* AND SELF-INDULGENCE

Hedonism is the pursuit of, or devotion to, pleasure; the self-gratifying feeling it brings relies on dopaminergic nerve pathways and the psychological reward system in the brain. It is specifically these areas of the brain that deteriorate in Parkinson's patients, which explains their tendency experience anhedonia (the inability to feel pleasure), apathy, and depression.

In Parkinson's the "hedonic tone"[434] is decreased and the solution is to promote activities centered on joy and pleasure.[373] Any pleasant pastime will improve the patient's experience: even a video game will free up dopamine in the striatum.[275]

Excitement and pleasure improve the substantia nigra[175] And the most pleasureable and exciting therapy is sex (associated with love, if possible). Sexual experiences activate many important pathways in the deep structures of the brain.

4. FAMILY AND FRIENDS

A bad marriage exacerbates Parkinson's. The negative outlook of a stressed or afflicted conjugal relationship worsens the effects of the disease.[184] The same occurs with other relatives and friendships.[185] These psychological and psychosocial aspects are now considered to be important factors in discerning the level of intensity of Parkinson's symptoms[185] and possibly its pathology as well.

Parkinson's symptoms are expressed in various ways depending on family and conjugal interactions.[217, 353, 548] It is necessary to avoid stressful emotional experiences.[138]

Parkinson's patients who perform worse are those who do not take advantage of social and family supports, and who face the disease with an excessively belligerent approach ("fight mode"), with a depressive attitude of giving in to defeat, or by taking an evasive stance.[36, 194]

5. MANAGING EMOTIONS

There is a failure of the emotional process in Parkinson's patients. It is observed in the phenomenon of *kinesia paradoxa* (in which the patient cannot move, but under certain emotional circumstances exhibits a sudden, brief period of mobility); and is due to disorders of the nuclei and underlying pathways. The amygdala in the brain modulates emotional responses; it absorbs less dopamine if medication is taken away, and is normalized with levodopa.[553]

Adverse emotional responses or negative thoughts increase motor freezing and are ameliorated by relaxation.[321]

Some Parkinson's patients become addicted to gambling and their preferred game is the slot machine. Interestingly, this emotional/behavioral deviation only occurs during an *on* period, in patients on levodopa, and it acts on previously damaged pathways in the brain.[376]

In light of all this, psychotherapy should be oriented to favor good emotional hygiene: it should involve a plan for eliminating negative thinking and dispelling hostility and inflexible attitudes. It should be understood that anger and intolerance are harmful and staying in a good mood should be part of the treatment program.

DISCARDING NEGATIVITY

Our kidneys expel toxic substances by urination, and our intestines do away with useless or harmful substances in the form of feces. In the same way, our brain should act to dispel the effects of negativity and help us avoid people who contaminate our emotional sphere. We should to flee from unhappy, demanding people and anyone who provokes bad feelings.

A patient who was a university professor was required to attend a dinner that would include the dean and some colleagues with whom he did not get on well. Anticipation of this event caused him to tremble and freeze up. I had recommended that he increase his dose of Sinemet before the social event, and later I realized my mistake: if he would rather watch a football game with real friends or take his family to the beach, by all means do it. Is this not a better alternative to taking extra pills to just be miserable? I told him to write his own social biography rather than pad his "social resume". This may not help him climb the professional ladder, but his neurons with thank him.

ET COLE FELICES, MISERO FUGE

"Select the lucky and avoid the unlucky" is the advice of the philosopher Baltasar Gracián.

In life, like in cards, the trick to know how to get rid of the bad cards. "You need to cut ties with those who contaminate your life," this is a prescription for selfishness. I wrote these words in 1997, in the first edition of my book *The Strange Case of Dr. Parkinson*. I put them in a controversial chapter about "unorthodox treatments". I now consider this a fundamental therapy.

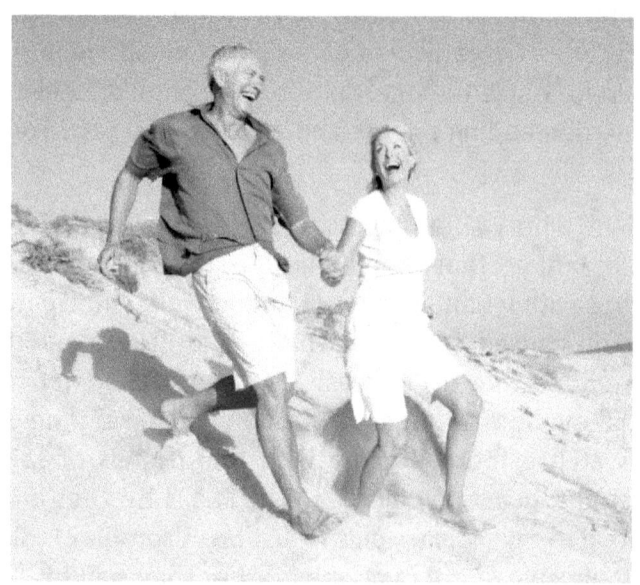

Exercise and physical activity, especially outdoors, is the best natural treatment for Parkinson's disease.

It relieves muscles and joints, frees up endorphins, relaxes, increases dopamine and promotes neuronal plasticity.

IX. Exercise and Fresh Air

There are two types of Parkinson's patients: those who live poorly and die early[280] (because all they do is take medicine), and those who live longer and better because they not only take pills, but they exercise.[161]

All Parkinson's patients are recommended to get physical therapy and rehabilitation. Few people heed this advice because they forget or because it is not explained clearly enough: exercise raises dopamine levels, relieves symptoms, protects neurons in the stratia nigra and constitutes the principal natural treatment for Parkinson's. It also has a preventive role: people who do intensive exercise in their youth show a lower risk of contracting Parkinson's.[506, 555]

Every Parkinsons's patient should exercise every day either in a rehabilitation center or with supervision: this will improve motor capacity, global functional capacity, memory, and other functions.[221] The best activity is a daily walk. For indoor options there are useful books[43, 82] and some valuable recommendations on the internet.[634]

DIRECT AND INDIRECT EFFECTS

Exercise has peripheral, or indirect, benefits: joints become more flexible, osteoporosis is avoided, and muscles are strengthened. There are also benefits directly related to Parkinson's: it rewires the motor pathways in the brain.

In Parkinson's, exercise increases dopamine levels the striatum,[408] improves symptoms,[627] promotes neuronal plasticity and neurogenesis,[346] and enhances motor control, decreasing the incidence of falling. It also helps avoid depression and sleep disorders. Taken as a whole, exercise provides is an increase in functional independence, a feeling of well-being and good quality of life.[34]

EXERCISE PROGRAM

A physical therapist can program the exercises adapted for each patient according to individual flexibility, strength, and cardiovascular capacity. A cardiologist's report would be needed.

The exercises are designed to improve coordination, balance, gait, and other movements, and are adapted for each particular case.[579]

The physical therapist should keep in mind that Parkinson's patients have special concerns regarding motor control deficit. For example, physical therapy should mainly address trunk movement and the wider ranges of motion, using a clave (percussive instrument) to achieve rhythmic motor patterns.[211]

FUNDAMENTALS

No one will dispute that exercise is good for the heart, and the same goes for the brain: physical activity prevents Parkinson's and other neurodegenerative disorders.[6, 7, 27, 412]

In reviewing eight studies of 144 Parkinson's patients, it was found that exercise promotes neuronal plasticity, the volume of grey matter, and the levels of neurotrophic factors.[208] There is evidence that exercise improves Parkinson's patients' symptoms, mood, cognition, and sleep.[453] In treated patients, the concentrations of levodopa en the blood increases with exercise.[452]

A NEUROPROTECTIVE EFFECT IN ANIMALS

Physical activity is neuroprotective because it increases mitochondrial respiration, antioxidant responses, and neuroplasticity. This has been shown in mice with MPTP and 6-OHDP-induced parkonsonism: animals that were previously subjected to exercise were protected and experienced less dopaminergic neuron loss and fewer motor and behavioral disorders.[558, 566, 627]

In animal models, *in vitro* as well as *in vivo*, exercise improves cognition and neuroplasticity, strengthens neurotrophic factors, more so if the exercise is vigorous.[6]

In mice with MPTP-induced chronic parkinsonism, sedentary patients were compared with those who were required to exercise on a wheel for 18 months. The latter showed greater mobility and coordination, improvement in mitochondria function and increased levels of dopamine and neurotrophic factors.[285]

FLEXIBILITY OF THE SPINE

Functional limitations of Parkinson's patients depends to a large degree on the flexibility of the spinal column. There are special exercise programs for the spine in which the patient follows a movement pattern designed to promote flexibility: the patient starts in a supine position and is taught, in successive phases, to arrive at a sitting position and, later, to stand. Axial stiffness is progressively relieved, unhealthy posture is discouraged, and bed-related movements become easier.[492]

SPORTS LEARNED IN YOUTH

In terms of sports, the focus should be on those the patients have already practiced to avoid the difficulty of learning new ones. The most appropriate sports for Parkinsons's patients are swimming (for those who already know how), hiking and gymnastics.[154]

HIPPOTHERAPY: HORSEBACK RIDING

Hippus is Greek for horse. Hippotherapy is treatment based on horseback riding for osteomuscular pathologies and coordination. The horse acts as an intermediary for motor impulses thereby contributing, by means of its activity, to the relaxation, strengthening, and adjustment of the locomotor apparatus.

Riding requires the musculature to constantly readapt to the movement of the horse's back, and this provides the effects of readjusting the rider's vertebrae and improving motor coordination, along with the added benefit of physical and psychological relaxation.[209]

It could benefit Parkinson's patients in the early stages as long as they work with a specialized physiotherapist, a well-trained horse, and a fully trained therapeutic assistant.

RESISTANCE TRAINING

Parkinson's patients with mild to moderate symptoms should build strength and physical performance in the same way (and with more reason) as healthy people of the same age. They need an athletic training and resistance program designed to increase strength, flexibility and coordination.[451, 489]

Fourteen Parkinson's patients with mild to moderate symptoms who were required to do resistance training for eight weeks saw an improvement in their gait and in their overall functional ability..[489] Using a different intensive training program that included aquatic exercise over a period of 14 weeks, a distinct improvement was found: surprisingly, even dyskinesias improved.[451]

MOUNTAIN HIKES

Nineteen Parkinson's patients participated in a week-long program of short hikes (from 3 to 6 kilometers) daily over mountainous terrain, and social gatherings and functions were included. The benefits were evident within a week, with obvious improvements in terms of their Parkinson's disease, but the benefits were short-lived: a revision four months later showed that they had regressed to their original states. Nevertheless, it is clear that it is beneficial to work out in a mountain environment that offers new situations and visual cues.[313]

AEROBICS

Aerobics is a physical training method meant to increase the body's oxygen intake. Typical aerobic exercises (walking, running, dancing, swimming, bicycling, etc.) stimulate cardiac and pulmonary activity enough to produce beneficial effects for the body, while building muscle strength at the same time. Aerobic training requires at least three sessions per week. In each session, the heart rate should be raised to the appropriate training level for a period of at least 20 minutes.

In healthy people, and more so for Parkinson's patients, aerobic exercise reduces stress, improves mood, increases physical ability and reduces fatigue. In controlled studies of aerobic exercise (16 weeks) with Parkinson's patients, not only was there a 26% improvement in lung capacity (this also occurs in normal subjects), but hypokinesia and freezing episodes were improved: reaction time for movement was reduced as much for simple movements as for specialized ones.[45] It is important to remember that aerobic exercise may be contraindicated in some older patients or those with heart problems.

BIKES

It is not only children and teens who benefit from riding bikes. In the autumn of our lives (and winter too) bicycles or motorcycles develop neural pathways which can atrophy in people who prefer the safety of four wheeled transportation. Remember those slim older persons who were physically and mentally agile who chose bikes as their means of transport throughout their lives. Over the years, not only do the benefit from the basic physical activity, but they develop webs of nerves and muscles that integrate balance and visual and spacial perception. It is a method of psychomotor rehabilitation with a special focus on the brain circuitry involving balance.

The best present for one's children (or grandchildren) is a bicycle. The rhythm of pedaling is especially helpful in preventing Parkinson's or alleviating its symptoms. We know that all exercise raises dopamine levels, but it is the act of pedaling, the continual balancing action, the sun and fresh air in one's face, the visual rewards while riding... it all creates a feast of sensory input for the basal nuclei and the cerebral cortex, and for the entire nervous system.

"Forced" pedaling (a mode of exercise in which a participant's voluntary rate is augmented on a stationary cycle) is even more beneficial as has been demonstrated in functional connectivity MRI studies. The technology of fMRI (functional magnetic resonance) is advancing rapidly and offers the possibility of directly measuring brain activity and connectivity in Parkinson's patients[554] using markers that allow researchers to detect changes in the substancia nigra or the cortex.[437] In a study of 27 patients that were made to pedal a stationary bicycle for 8 weeks at either their voluntary rate or a forced rate, functional connectivity was found to increase in line with pedaling rate. This shows that an increase in the rate of pedaling improves thalamocortical connectivity.[501] Other studies have also shown that vigorous activity is quite effective,[6, 540] relieving stiffness, improving gait, temblor and dyskinesias, and can prove to be a useful therapy.[540]

FRESH AIR AND SUNSHINE

I need to feel the sun on my face before breakfast. As well as generating vitamin D, going out in the sun and fresh air, among nature or in the street, we obtain several benefits: the exercise of walking and the sensory nutrition of being outdoors.

Exercise is even more beneficial when done outdoors. Being outside is healing: it is good for Parkinson's patients to see people and storefronts as they walk. It is even better to stroll on the beach, barefoot in the sand, smelling the sea with the sun and breeze caressing one's face. It is a diet of sunlight, wind, and life.

PLEASURE, MUSCLES, AND THE MIND

Physical activity is a great way of relieving tension. When we exercise, we secrete endorphins, natural tranquilizers that relax the body physiologically allowing the muscles to strengthen and stretch. This stretching promotes joint mobility.

Physical exercise, when seen as pleasure and recreation, is another way of transferring to the body some elements that uplift mood: energy, audacity, and patience. The exercise could be swimming, walking, or normal or stationary biking. Whatever it is, physical activity, especially when done outdoors, is the best natural treatment for Parkinson's disease.

5

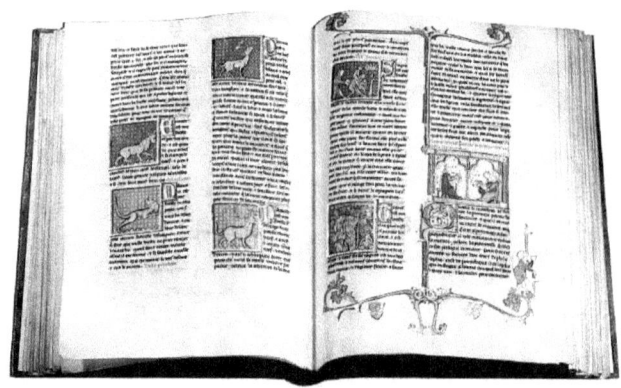

The book contains **636 bibliographic references** of scientific interest.

Bibliography

1. Abbott RA, Cox M, Markus H, Tomkins A. Diet, body size and micronutrient status in Parkinson's disease. Eur J Clin Nutr 1992; 46:879-884.

2. Aguiar S, Borowski T. Neuropharmacological review of the nootropic herb Bacopa monnieri. Rejuvenation Res. 2013 Aug;16(4):313-26.

3. Aguilar M, Romero S, Molina-Porcel L, Pastor P. Significant improvement of adult-onset dystonia with cannabinoidsbased oromucosal spray. 20th International Congress of Parkinson's Disease and Movement Disorders. Berlin, 2016. Movement Disorders 2016; 31 (Suppl 2):S695-696.

4. Ahlemeyer B, Krieglstein J. Pharmacological studies supporting the therapeutic use of Ginkgo biloba extract for Alzheimer's disease. Pharmacopsychiatry. 2003 Jun;36 Suppl 1:S8-14.

5. Ahlemeyer B, Krieglstein J. Neuroprotective effects of Ginkgo biloba extract. Cell Mol Life Sci. 2003 Sep;60(9):1779-92.

6. Ahlskog JE. Does vigorous exercise have a neuroprotective effect in Parkinson disease? Neurology. 2011 Jul 19;77(3):288-94.

7. Ahlskog JE, Geda YE, Graff-Radford NR, Petersen RC. Physical exercise as a preventive or disease-modifying treatment of dementia and brain aging. Mayo Clin Proc. 2011 Sep;86(9):876-84.

8. Ahmad B, Lapidus LJ. Curcumin prevents aggregation in alfa-synuclein by increasing reconfiguration rate. J Biol Chem. 2012 Mar 16;287(12):9193-9.

9. Ahmad M, Saleem S, Ahmad AS., et al. Ginkgo biloba affords dose-dependent protection against 6-hydroxydopamine-induced parkinsonism in rats: neurobehavioural, neurochemical and immuno-histochemical evidences. J Neurochem. 2005; 93(1): 94–104.

10. Ahmed I, John A, Vijayasarathy C, Robin MA, Raza H. Differential modulation of growth and glutathione metabolism in cultured rat astrocytes by 4-hydroxy-nonenal and green tea polyphenol, epigallocatechin-3-gallate. Neurotoxicology 2002; 23:289-300.

11. Airola P. How to get well. Health Plus Publishers, Phoenix 1988.

12. Akhondzadeh S, Kashani L, Mobaseri M, Hosseini SH, Nikzad S, Khani M. Passionflower in the treatment of opiates withdrawal: a double-blind randomized controlled trial. J Clin Pharm Ther. 2001 Oct;26(5):369-73. (a)

13. Akhondzadeh S, Naghavi HR, Vazirian M, Shayeganpour A, Rashidi H, Khani M. Passionflower in the treatment of generalized anxiety: a pilot double-blind randomized controlled trial with oxazepam. J Clin Pharm Ther 2001; 26:363-367. (b)

14. Albani D, Polito L, Forloni G. Sirtuins as novel targets for Alzheimer's disease and other neurodegenerative disorders: experimental and genetic evidence. J Alzheimers Dis. 2010;19(1):11-26.

15. Albani D, Polito L, Signorini A, Forloni G. Neuroprotective properties of resveratrol in different neurodegenerative disorders. Biofactors. 2010 Sep-Oct;36(5):370-6.

16. Alcalay RN, Gu Y, Mejia-Santana H, Cote L, Marder KS, Scarmeas N. The association between Mediterranean diet adherence and Parkinson's disease. Mov Disord. 2012 May;27(6):771-4.

17. Al-Karawi D, Al Mamoori DA, Tayyar Y. The Role of Curcumin Administration in Patients with Major Depressive Disorder: Mini Meta-Analysis of Clinical Trials. Phytother Res. 2016 Feb;30(2):175-83.

18. Ameri A. The effects of cannabinoids on the brain. Prog Neurobiol 1999; 58:315-348.

19. Amieva H, Meillon C, Helmer C, Barberger-Gateau P, Dartigues JF. Ginkgo biloba extract and long-term cognitive decline: a 20-year follow-up population-based study. PLoS One. 2013;8(1):e52755

20. Anandhan A, Tamilselvam K, Vijayraja D, Ashokkumar N, Rajasankar S, Manivasagam T. Resveratrol attenuates oxidative stress and improves behaviour in 1 -methyl-4-phenyl-1,2,3,6-tetrahydropyridine (MPTP) challenged mice. Ann Neurosci. 2010 Jul;17(3):113-9.

21. Anderson C, Checkoway H, Franklin GM, Beresford S, Smith-Weller T, Swanson PD. Dietary factors in Parkinson's disease: the role of food groups and specific foods. Mov Disord 1999; 14:21-27.

22. Andres K, Bellwald L, Brenner HD. [Empirical study of physically orientated therapy with schizophrenic patients]. Z Klin Psychol Psycopathol Psychother 1993; 41:159-169

23. Anonymous. EGb 761: ginkgo biloba extract, Ginkor. Drugs R D. 2003;4(3):188-93.

24. Apaydin H, Ertan S, Ozekmekci S. Broad bean (Vicia faba) -a natural source of L-dopa- prolongs "on" periods in patients with Parkinson's disease who have "on-off" fluctuations. Mov Disord 2000; 15:164-166.

25. Appel K, Rose T, Fiebich B, Kammler T, Hoffmann C, Weiss G. Modulation of the ?-aminobutyric acid (GABA) system by Passiflora incarnata L. Phytother Res. 2011 Jun;25(6):838-43.

26. Arad S, Bar-Lev Schleider L, Knaani J, Shabtai H, Balash Y, Ezra A, Giladi N, Gurevich T. Medical cannabis for the treatment of Tourette syndrome: A descriptive analysis of 24 patients. 20th International Congress of Parkinson's Disease and Movement Disorders. Berlin, 2016. Movement Disorders 2016; 31 (Suppl 2):S309-S310.

27. Arnao V, Di Raimondo D, Tuttolomondo A, Pinto A. Neurotrophic and Neuroprotective effects of muscle contraction. Curr Pharm Des. 2016 Apr 28. [Epub ahead of print]

28. Ascherio A, Zhang SM, Hernan MA, Kawachi I, Colditz GA, Speizer FE, Willett WC. Prospective study of caffeine consumption and risk of Parkinson's disease in men and women. Ann Neurol 2001; 50:56-63

29. Ashraf W, Pfeiffer RF, Park F, et al. Constipation in Parkinson's disease: objective assessment and response to psyllium. Mov Disord 1997; 12:946–51.

30. Aslanargun P1, Cuvas O, Dikmen B, Aslan E, Yuksel MU. Passiflora incarnata Linneaus as an anxiolytic before spinal anesthesia. J Anesth. 2012 Feb;26(1):39-44.

31. Astarloa R, Mena MA, Sanchez V, de la Vega L, de Yebenes JG. Clinical and pharmacokinetic effects of a diet rich in insoluble fiber on Parkinson disease. Clin Neuropharmacol 1992; 15:375-380.

32. Augustin AD1,2, Charlett A1,3, Weller C1, Dobbs SM1,2,4, Taylor D1,2, Bjarnason I4, Dobbs RJ1,2,4. Quantifying rigidity of Parkinson's disease in relation to laxative treatment: a service evaluation. Br J Clin Pharmacol 2016 Apr 8.

33. Avery A. Aromatherapy and you.Blue Heron Hill Press, Kailua, HI 1992.

34. Baatile J, Langbein WE, Weaver F, Maloney C, Jost MB. Effect of exercise on perceived quality of life of individuals with Parkinson's disease. J Rehabil Res Dev 2000; 37:529-534.

35. Babu US, Wiesenfeld PW, Collins TF, Sprando R, Flynn TJ, Black T, Olejnik N, Raybourne RB. Impact of high flaxseed diet on mitogen-induced proliferation, IL-2 production, cell subsets and fatty acid composition of spleen cells from pregnant and F1 generation Sprague-Dawley rats. Food Chem Toxicol. 2003; 41:905-915

36. Backer JH. Stressors, social support, coping, and health dysfunction in individuals with Parkinson's disease. J Gerontol Nurs 2000;26:6-16.

37. Badia P, et al. 1990. Responsiveness to olfactory stimuli presented in sleep. Physiol Behavior 48: 87-90.

38. Bara-Jimenez W, Sherzai A, Dimitrova T, Favit A, Bibbiani F, Gillespie M, Morris MJ, Mouradian MM, Chase TN. Adenosine A(2A) receptor antagonist treatment of Parkinson's disease. Neurology. 2003 Aug 12;61(3):293-6.

39. Barboza JL, Okun MS2, Moshiree B3. The treatment of gastroparesis, constipation and small intestinal bacterial overgrowth syndrome in patients withParkinson's disease. Expert Opin Pharmacother. 2015;16(16):2449-64.

40. Barichella M, Marczewska A, Vairo A, Canesi M, Pezzoli G. Is underweightness still a major problem in Parkinson's disease patients? Eur J Clin Nutr 2003; 57:543-547.

41. Barranco Quintana JL, Allam MF, Del Castillo AS, Navajas RF. Parkinson's disease and tea: a quantitative review. J Am Coll Nutr. 2009 Feb;28(1):1-6.

42. Bastianetto S, Zheng WH, Quirion R. The Ginkgo biloba extract (EGb 761) protects and rescues hippocampal cells against nitric oxide-induced toxicity: involvement of its flavonoid constituents and protein kinase C. J Neurochem. 2000 Jun;74(6):2268-77.

43. Bayés Rusiañol A. Rehabilitación integral de la enfermedad de Parkinson y otros parkinsonismos. Ars medica, Barcelona 2002.

44. Benton D, Donohoe RT. The effects of nutrients on mood. Public Health Nutr 1999;2:403-9.

45. Bergen JL, Toole T, Elliott RG 3rd, Wallace B, Robinson K, Maitland CG. Aerobic exercise intervention improves aerobic capacity and movement initiation in Parkinson's disease patients. NeuroRehabilitation 2002; 17:161-168

46. Berry EM, Growdon JH, Wurtman JJ, Caballero B, Wurtman RJ. A balanced carbohydrate: protein diet in the management of Parkinson's disease. Neurology 1991; 41:1295-1297.

47. Bertoldi M, Gonsalvi M, Voltattorni CB. Green tea polyphenols: novel irreversible inhibitors of dopa decarboxylase. Biochem Biophys Res Commun. 2001 Jun 1;284(1):90-3.

48. Bia?ecka M, Kurzawski M, Roszmann A, Robowski P, Sitek EJ, Honczarenko K, Gorzkowska A, Budrewicz S, Mak M, Jarosz M, Go??b-Janowska M,Koziorowska-Gawron E, Dro?dzik M, S?awek J. Association of COMT, MTHFR, and SLC19A1(RFC-1) polymorphisms with homocysteine blood levels and cognitive impairment in Parkinson's disease. Pharmacogenet Genomics 2012; 22:716-24.

49. Birks J, Grimley Evans J. Ginkgo biloba for cognitive impairment and dementia. Cochrane Database Syst Rev. 2009 Jan 21;(1):CD003120.

50. Blanchet J, Longpré F, Bureau G, Morissette M, DiPaolo T, Bronchti G, Martinoli MG. Resveratrol, a red wine polyphenol, protects dopaminergic neurons in MPTP-treated mice. Prog Neuropsychopharmacol Biol Psychiatry. 2008 Jul 1;32(5):1243-50.

51. Bone KM. Potential interaction of Ginkgo biloba leaf with antiplatelet or anticoagulant drugs: what is the evidence? Mol Nutr Food Res. 2008 Jul;52(7):764-71.

52. Boniel T, Dannon P. [The safety of herbal medicines in the psychiatric practice] Harefuah 2001; 140:780-805.

53. Bonnefoy M, Drai J, Kostka T. [Antioxidants to slow aging, facts and perspectives]. Presse Med 2002; 31:1174-1184

54. Bové J, Prou D, Perier C, Przedborski S. Toxin-Induced Models of Parkinson's Disease. NeuroRx. 2005 Jul; 2(3): 484–494.

55. Bracco F, Malesani R, Saladini M, Battistin L. Protein redistribution diet and antiparkinsonian response to levodopa. Eur Neurol 1991; 31:68-71.

56. Bradford N (ed). The Hamlyn Encyclopedia of Complementary Health. Reed International Books Ltd, London 1996.

57. Bridi R, Crossetti FP, Steffen VM, Henriques AT. The antioxidant activity of standardized extract of Ginkgo biloba (EGb 761) in rats. Phytother Res 2001; 15:449-451.

58. Broadley KJ, Akhtar Anwar M, Herbert AA, Fehler M, Jones EM, Davies WE, Kidd EJ, Ford WR. Effects of dietary amines on the gut and its vasculature. Br J Nutr. 2009 Jun;101(11):1645-52.

59. Brooker DJ, Snape M, Johnson E, Ward D, Payne M. Single case evaluation of the effects of aroma-therapy and massage on disturbed behaviour in severe dementia. Br J Clin Psychol 1997; 36:287-296.

60. Brotchie JM. Adjuncts to dopamine replacement: a pragmatic approach to reducing the problem of dyskinesia in Parkinson's disease. Mov Disord 1998; 13:871-876.

61. Brown E, Hurd NS, McCall S, Ceremuga TE. Evaluation of the anxiolytic effects of chrysin, a Passiflora incarnata extract, in the laboratory rat. AANA J. 2007 Oct;75(5):333-7.

62. Bruce-Keller AJ, Umberger G, McFall R, Mattson MP. Food restriction reduces brain damage and improves behavioral outcome following excitotoxic and metabolic insults. Ann Neurol 1999; 45:8-15.

63. Bruinsma K, Taren DL. Chocolate: food or drug? J Am Diet Assoc 1999; 99:1249-1256.

64. Buckle J. The smell of relief. Psychology today 2000; 33:24.

65. Buckley J. Massage and aromatherapy massage: nursing art and science. Int J Palliat Nurs 2002; 8:276-280.

66. Calder PC. Fatty acids and inflammation: the cutting edge between food and pharma. Eur J Pharmacol. 2011 Sep;668 Suppl 1:S50-8.

67. Calder PC. The role of marine omega-3 (n-3) fatty acids in inflammatory processes, atherosclerosis and plaque stability. Mol Nutr Food Res. 2012 Jul;56(7):1073-80.

68. Calderón-Garcidueñas L, Mora-Tiscareño A, Franco-Lira M, Cross JV, Engle R, Aragón-Flores M, Gómez-Garza G, Jewells V, Medina-Cortina H, Solorio E, Chao CK, Zhu H, Mukherjee PS, Ferreira-Azevedo L, Torres-Jardón R,D'Angiulli A. Flavonol-rich dark cocoa significantly decreases plasma endothelin-1 and improves cognition in urban children. Front Pharmacol. 2013 Aug 22;4:104.

69. Calenda E, Weinstein S. Therapeutic massage. En: Weintraub MI (ed.) Alternative and complementary treatment in neurologic illness. Churchill Livingstone, New York 2001.

70. Camicioli RM, Bouchard TP, Somerville MJ. Homocysteine is not associated with global motor or cognitive measures in nondemented older Parkinson's disease patients. Mov Disord. 2009 Jan 30;24(2):176-82.

71. Cao F, Sun S, Tong ET. Experimental study on inhibition of neuronal toxical effect of levodopa by ginkgo biloba extract on Parkinson disease in rats. J Huazhong Univ Sci Technolog Med Sci. 2003;23:151-3.

72. Caparros-Lefebvre D, Elbaz A. Possible relation of atypical parkinsonism in the French West Indies with consumption of tropical plants: a case-control study. Caribbean Parkinsonism Study Group. Lancet 1999; 354:281-286.

73. Caporael LR. Ergotism: The Satan loosed in Salem? Science 1976; 192: 21-26.

74. Cardoso HD, dos Santos Junior EF, de Santana DF, Gonçalves-Pimentel C, Angelim MK, Isaac AR,Lagranha CJ, Guedes RC, Beltrão EI, Morya E, Rodrigues MC, Andrade-da-Costa BL. Omega-3 deficiency and neurodegeneration in the substantia nigra: involvement of increased nitric oxide production and reduced BDNF expression. Biochim Biophys Acta. 2014 Jun;1840(6):1902-12.

75. Cardoso HD, Passos PP, Lagranha CJ, Ferraz AC, Santos Júnior EF, Oliveira RS, Oliveira PE, Santos Rde C, Santana DF, Borba JM, Rocha-de-Melo AP,Guedes RC, Navarro DM, Santos GK, Borner R, Picanço-Diniz CW, Beltrão EI, Silva JF, Rodrigues MC, Andrade da Costa BL. Differential vulnerability of substantia nigra and corpus striatum to oxidative insult induced by reduced dietary levels of essential fatty acids. Front Hum Neurosci. 2012 Aug 30;6:249.

76. Carod-Artal FJ. Síndromes neurológicos asociados con el consumo de plantas y hongos con componente tóxico (I). Síndromes neurotóxicos causados por la ingestión de plantas, semillas y frutos. Rev Neurol 2003; 36:860-871.

77. Carod-Artal FJ. Síndromes neurológicos asociados con el consumo de plantas y hongos con componente tóxico (II). Hongos y plantas alucinógenos, micotoxinas y hierbas medicinales. Rev Neurol 2003; 36:951-960.

78. Carter JH, Nutt JG, Woodward WR, Hatcher LF, Trotman TL. Amount and distribution of dietary protein affects clinical response to levodopa in Parkinson's disease. Neurology 1989; 39:552-556

79. Caruana M, Vassallo N. Tea Polyphenols in Parkinson's Disease. Adv Exp Med Biol. 2015;863:117-37.

80. Cash AH; el-Mallakh RS; Chamberlain K; Bratton JZ; Li R. Structure of music may influence cognition. Percept Mot Skills 1997; 84:66.

81. Caso Marasco A, Vargas Ruiz R, Salas Villa-gomez A, Begona Infante C. Estudio doble ciego sobre complejo multivitamínico suplementado con extracto estandarizado de Ginseng. Drugs Exp Clin Res 1996; 22: 323-329.

82. Castro García A, López del Val LJ. La enfermedad de Parkinson y la vida cotidiana. Ergón, Madrid 1998.

83. Ceravolo R, Cossu G, Bandettini di Poggio M, Santoro L, Barone P, Zibetti M, Frosini D, Nicoletti V, Manganelli F, Iodice R, Picillo M, Merola A, Lopiano L,Paribello A, Manca D, Melis M, Marchese R, Borelli P, Mereu A, Contu P, Abbruzzese G, Bonuccelli U. Neuropathy and levodopa in Parkinson's disease: evidence from a multicenter study. Mov Disord. 2013 Sep;28(10):1391-7.

84. Chagas MH, Eckeli AL, Zuardi AW, Pena-Pereira MA, Sobreira-Neto MA, Sobreira ET, Camilo MR, Bergamaschi MM, Schenck CH, Hallak JE, Tumas V,Crippa JA. Cannabidiol can improve complex sleep-related behaviours associated with rapid eye movement sleep behaviour disorder in Parkinson's disease patients: a case series. J Clin Pharm Ther. 2014 Oct;39(5):564-6.

85. Chagas MH, Zuardi AW, Tumas V, Pena-Pereira MA, Sobreira ET, Bergamaschi MM, dos Santos AC, Teixeira AL, Hallak JE, Crippa JA. Effects of cannabidiol in the treatment of patients with Parkinson's disease: an exploratory double-blind trial. J Psychopharmacol. 2014;28:1088-98.

86. Chan AL, Leung HW, Wu JW, Chien TW. Risk of hemorrhage associated with co-prescriptions for Ginkgo biloba and antiplatelet or anticoagulant drugs. J Altern Complement Med 2011;17:513-7.

87. Chan DK, Woo J, Ho SC, Pang CP, Law LK, Ng PW, Hung WT, Kwok T, Hui E, Orr K, Leung MF, Kay R. Genetic and environmental risk factors for Parkinson's disease in a Chinese population. J Neurol Neurosurg Psychiatry 1998; 65:781-784

88. Chang LC, Huang N, Chou YJ, Kao FY, Hsieh PC, Huang YT. Patterns of combined prescriptions of aspirin-Ginkgo biloba in Taiwan: a population-based study. J Clin Pharm Ther. 2008 Jun;33(3):243-9.

89. Chao J, Yu MS, Ho YS, Wang M, Chang RC. Dietary oxyresveratrol prevents parkinsonian mimetic 6-hydroxydopamine neurotoxicity. Free Radic Biol Med. 2008 Oct 1;45(7):1019-26.

90. Chaperon F, Thiebot MH. Behavioral effects of cannabinoid agents in animals. Crit Rev Neurobiol 1999; 13:243-281.

91. Checkoway H, Powers K, Smith-Weller T, Franklin GM, Longstreth WT Jr, Swanson PD. Parkinson's disease risks associated with cigarette smoking, alcohol consumption, and caffeine intake. Am J Epidemiol 2002; 155:732-738

92. Cheesman S, Christian R, Cresswell J. Exploring the value of shiatsu in palliative care day services. Int J Palliat Nurs 2001; 7:234-239.

93. Chen CF, Chiou WF, Zhang JT. Comparison of the pharmacological effects of Panax ginseng and Panax quinquefolium. Acta Pharmacol Sin. 2008 Sep;29(9):1103-8.

94. Chen WW, Cheng X, Zhang X, Zhang QS, Sun HQ, Huang WJ, Xie ZY. The expression features of serum Cystatin C and homocysteine of Parkinson's disease with mild cognitive dysfunction. Eur Rev Med Pharmacol Sci. 2015 Aug;19(16):2957-63.

95. Chen XC, Zhou YC, Chen Y, Zhu YG, Fang F, Chen LM. Ginsenoside Rg1 reduces MPTP-induced substantia nigra neuron loss by suppressing oxidative stress. Acta Pharmacol Sin. 2005 Jan;26:56-62.

96. Cherkin DC, Sherman KJ, Deyo RA, Shekelle PG. A review of the evidence for the effectiveness, safety, and cost of acupuncture, massage therapy, and spinal manipulation for back pain. Ann Intern Med. 2003 Jun 3;138(11):898-906.

97. Cho IH. Effects of Panax ginseng in Neurodegenerative Diseases. J Ginseng Res 2012;36:342-53.

98. Choi JY, Park CS, Kim DJ, Cho MH, Jin BK, Pie JE, Chung WG. Prevention of nitric oxide-mediated 1-methyl-4-phenyl-1,2,3,6-tetrahydropyridine-induced Parkinson's disease in mice by tea phenolic epigallocatechin 3-gallate. Neurotoxicology 2002; 23: 367-374

99. Choi S, Jung SY, Lee JH, Sala F, Criado M, Mulet J, Valor LM, Sala S, Engel AG, Nah SY. Effects of ginsenosides, active components of ginseng, on nicotinic acetylcholine receptors expressed in Xenopus oocytes. Eur J Pharmacol 2002; 442:37-45.

100. Churchill JD, Gerson JL, Hinton KA, Mifek JL, Walter MJ, Winslow CL, Deyo RA. The nootropic properties of ginseng saponin Rb1 are linked to effects on anxiety. Integr Physiol Behav Sci 2002; 37: 178-187.

101. Coon JT, Ernst E. Panax ginseng: a systematic review of adverse effects and drug interactions. Drug Saf 2002; 25:323-344.

102. Conrad GD. Is ginkgo biloba and/or a multivitamin-multimineral supplement a therapeutic option for Parkinson's disease? A case report. Glob Adv Health Med. 2014 Jul;3(4):43-4.

103. Coulombe K, Saint-Pierre M, Cisbani G, St-Amour I, Gibrat C, Giguère-Rancourt A, Calon F, Cicchetti F. Partial neurorescue effects of DHA following a 6-OHDA lesion of the mouse dopaminergic system. J Nutr Biochem. 2016 Apr;30:133-42.

104. Cox PA, Sacks OW. Cycad neurotoxins, consumption of flying foxes, and ALS-PDC disease in Guam. Neurology 2002; 58: 956-9.

105. Cullen L, Barlow J. 'Kiss, cuddle, squeeze': the experiences and meaning of touch among parents of children with autism attending a Touch Therapy Programme. J Child Health Care 2002; 6:171-181.

106. da Rocha Lindner G, Bonfanti Santos D, Colle D, Gasnhar Moreira EL, Daniel Prediger R, Farina M, Khalil NM,Mara Mainardes R. Improved neuroprotective effects of resveratrol-loaded polysorbate 80-coated poly(lactide) nanoparticles in MPTP-induced Parkinsonism. Nanomedicine 2015; 10:1127-38.

107. Dartigues JF, Carcaillon L, Helmer C, Lechevallier N, Lafuma A, Khoshnood B. Vasodilators and nootropics as predictors of dementia and mortality in the PAQUID cohort. J Am Geriatr Soc 2007; 55:395-9.

108. Darvesh AS, Carroll RT, Bishayee A, Novotny NA, Geldenhuys WJ, Van der Schyf CJ. Curcumin and neurodegenerative diseases: a perspective. Expert Opin Investig Drugs. 2012 Aug;21(8):1123-40. doi: 10.1517/13543784.2012.693479. Epub 2012 Jun 6.

109. Das A, Shanker G, Nath C, Pal R, Singh S, Singh H. A comparative study in rodents of standardized extracts of Bacopa monniera and Ginkgo biloba: anticholinesterase and cognitive enhancing activities. Pharmacol Biochem Behav. 2002 Nov;73(4):893-900.

110. de Castro-Neto EF, da Cunha RH, da Silveira DX, Yonamine M, Gouveia TL, Cavalheiro EA, Amado D, Naffah-Mazzacoratti Mda G. Changes in aminoacidergic and monoaminergic neurotransmission in the hippocampus and amygdala of rats after ayahuasca ingestion. World J Biol Chem. 2013 Nov 26;4(4):141-7.

111. DeFeudis FV, Drieu K. Ginkgo biloba extract (EGb 761) and CNS functions: basic studies and clinical applications. Curr Drug Targets. 2000 Jul;1(1):25-58.

112. de la Torre R, de Sola S, Hernandez G, Farré M, Pujol J, Rodriguez J, Espadaler JM, Langohr K, Cuenca-Royo A, Principe A, Xicota L, Janel N, Catuara-Solarz S, Sanchez-Benavides G, Bléhaut H, Dueñas-Espín I, Del Hoyo L, Benejam B, Blanco-Hinojo L, Videla S, Fitó M, Delabar JM, Dierssen M; TESDAD study group. Safety and efficacy of cognitive training plus epigallocatechin-3-gallate in young adults with Down's syndrome (TESDAD): a double-blind, randomised, placebo-controlled, phase 2 trial. Lancet Neurol. 2016 Jul;15(8):801-10.

113. de Oliveira RM, Pais TF, Outeiro TF. Sirtuins: common targets in aging and in neurodegeneration. Curr Drug Targets. 2010 Oct;11(10):1270-80.

114. Dergal JM, Gold JL, Laxer DA, Lee MS, Binns MA, Lanctot KL, Freedman M, Rochon PA. Potential interactions between herbal medicines and conven-tional drug therapies used by older adults attending a memory clinic. Drugs Aging 2002; 19:879-886.

115. Der Giessen RV, Olanow W, Lees A, Wagner H. Method for preparing Mucuna pruriens see extract. United States Patent, US 7,470,441 B2, Dec. 30, 2008.

116. Deyama T, Nishibe S, Nakazawa Y. Constituents and pharmacological effects of Eucommia and Siberian ginseng. Acta Pharmacol Sin 2001; 22:1057-1070.

117. Dhawan K. Drug/substance reversal effects of a novel tri-substituted benzoflavone moiety (BZF) isolated from Passiflora incarnata Linn.--a brief perspective. Addict Biol. 2003 Dec;8(4):379-86.

118. Dhawan K, Kumar S, Sharma A. Anti-anxiety studies on extracts of Passiflora incarnata Linneaus. J Ethnopharmacol 2001; 78:165-170.

119. Dhawan K, Sharma A. Antitussive activity of the methanol extract of Passiflora incarnata leaves. Fitoterapia 2002; 73:397-399.a

120. Dhawan K, Kumar S, Sharma A. Anxiolytic activity of aerial and underground parts of Passiflora incarnata. Fitoterapia 2001; 72:922-926.

121. Dhawan K, Kumar S, Sharma A. Comparative anxiolytic activity profile of various preparations of Passiflora incarnata linneaus: a comment on medicinal plants' standardization. J Altern Complement Med 2002; 8:283-291.b

122. Dhawan K, Kumar S, Sharma A. Reversal of cannabinoids (delta9-THC) by the benzoflavone moiety from methanol extract of Passiflora incarnata Linneaus in mice: a possible therapy for cannabinoid addiction. J Pharm Pharmacol. 2002 Jun;54(6):875-81. (C)

123. Diamond BJ, Shiflett SC, Feiwel N, Matheis RJ, Noskin O, Richards JA, Schoenberger NE. Ginkgo biloba extract: mechanisms and clinical indications. Arch Phys Med Rehabil. 2000;81:668-78.

124. Diego MA, Field T, Hernandez-Reif M, Shaw JA, Rothe EM, Castellanos D, Mesner L. Aggressive adolescents benefit from massage therapy. Adoles-cence 2002; 37:597-607.

125. Di Marzo, Bisogno T, De Petrocellis L. Endocannabinoids: new targets for drug development. Curr Pharm Des 2000; 6:1361-1380

126. Donoyama N, Suoh S, Ohkoshi N. Effectiveness of Anma massage therapy in alleviating physical symptoms in outpatients with Parkinson's disease: a before-after study. Complement Ther Clin Pract 2014 Nov;20(4):251-61.

127. dos Santos EF, Busanello EN, Miglioranza A, Zanatta A, Barchak AG, Vargas CR, Saute J, Rosa C, Carrion MJ, Camargo D, Dalbem A, da Costa JC, de Sousa Miguel SR, de Mello Rieder CR, Wajner M. Evidence that folic acid deficiency is a major determinant of hyperhomocysteinemia in Parkinson's disease. Metab Brain Dis. 2009 Jun;24(2):257-69.

128. Dos Santos KC, Borges TV, Olescowicz G, Ludka FK, Santos CA, Molz S. Passiflora actinia hydroalcoholic extract and its major constituent, isovitexin, are neuroprotective against glutamate-induced cell damage in mice hippocampal slices. J Pharm Pharmacol. 2016 Feb;68(2):282-91.

129. Dos Santos RG, Osório FL, Crippa JA, Hallak JE. Antidepressive and anxiolytic effects of ayahuasca: a systematic literature review of animal and human studies. Rev Bras Psquiatr 2016; 38:65-72.

130. Dror Y, Stern F, Berner YN, Kaufmann NA, Berry E, Maaravi Y, Altman H, Cohen A, Leventhal A, Kaluski DN. [Micronutrient (vitamins and minerals) supple-mentation for the elderly, suggested by a special committee nominated by Ministry of Health]. Harefuah 2001; 140:1062-7, 1117.

131. Du XX, Xu HM, Jiang H, Song N, Wang J, Xie JX.. Curcumin protects nigral dopaminergic neurons by iron-chelation in the 6-hydroxydopamine rat model of Parkinson's disease. Neurosci Bull 2012; 28:253-8.

132. Duan W, Ladenheim B, Cutler RG, Kruman II, Cadet JL, Mattson MP. Dietary folate deficiency and elevated homocysteine levels endanger dopaminergic neurons in models of Parkinson's disease. J Neurochemistry 2002; 80:101-110.

133. Duan W, Mattson MP. Dietary restriction and 2-deoxyglucose administration improve behavioral outcome and reduce degeneration of dopaminergic neurons in models of Parkinson's disease. J Neurosci Res 1999; 57:195-206.

134. Duke JA. The green pharmacy. Radale Press, Emaus 1997.

135. Durlach PJ. The effects of a low dose of caffeine on cognitive performance. Psychopharmacology (Berl) 1998; 140:116-119.

136. Dutta D, Mohanakumar KP. Tea and Parkinson's disease: Constituents of tea synergize with antiparkinsonian drugs to provide better therapeutic benefits. Neurochem Int. 2015 Oct;89:181-90.

137. Edwards, L. 1994. Aromatherapy and essential oils. Healthy and Natural Journal, Oct, 134-137.

138. Ellgring H, Seiler S, Perleth B, Frings W, Gasser T, Oertel W. Psychosocial aspects of Parkinson's disease. Neurology. 1993 Dec;43(12 Suppl 6):S41-4.

139. Elphick MR, Egertova M. The neurobiology and evolution of cannabinoid signalling. Philos Trans R Soc Lond B Biol Sci 2001 Mar 29;356(1407):381-408

140. Ellis JM, Reddy P. Effects of Panax ginseng on quality of life. Ann Pharmacother 2002; 36:375-379.

141. Engelberg D, McCutcheon A, Wiseman S. A case of ginseng-induced mania. J Clin Psychopharmacol 2001 Oct;21(5):535-7.

142. Ernst E. The risk-benefit profile of commonly used herbal therapies: Ginkgo, St. John's Wort, Ginseng, Echinacea, Saw Palmetto, and Kava. Ann Intern Med 2002;136:42-53.

143. Esin RG, Naprienko MV, Mukhametova ER, Khairullin IK, Esin OR. [Tanakan as a multimodal cytoprotective factor in general medicine (II)]. Zh Nevrol Psikhiatr Im S S Korsalova 2015; 115:177-82.

144. Fall PA, Fredrikson M, Axelson O, Granerus AK. Nutritional and occupational factors influencing the risk of Parkinson's disease: a case-control study in southeastern Sweden. Mov Disord 1999; 14:28-37.

145. Farlow M. A clinical overview of cholinesterase inhibitors in Alzheimer's disease. Int Psychogeriatr. 2002;14 Suppl 1:93-126.

146. Farr T, Nottle C, Nosaka K, Sacco P. The effects of therapeutic massage on delayed onset muscle soreness and muscle function following downhill walking. J Sci Med Sport. 2002 Dec;5(4):297-306.

147. Farre Albaladejo M. Complicaciones neurológicas de la drogadicción. Aspectos generales. Complicaciones producidas por cannabis, drogas de diseño y substancias volátiles. Arch Neurobiol (Madr) 1989; 52 (Suppl 1):143-148.

148. Favaro VM, Yonamine M, Soares JC, Oliveira MG. Effects of long-term ayahuasca administration on memory and anxiety in rats. PLoS One 2015;10:e0145840.

149. Feany MB, Bender WW. A Drosophila model of Parkinson's disease. Nature 2000; 23;404(6776):394-8.

150. Fernandez N, Carriedo D, Sierra M, Diez MJ, Sahagun A, Calle A, Gonzalez A, Garcia JJ. Hydrosoluble fiber (Plantago ovata husk) and levodopa II: experimental study of the pharmacokinetic interaction in the presence of carbidopa. Eur Neuropsychopharmacol. 2005 Oct;15(5):505-9.

151. Fernández-Fernández L, Esteban G, Giralt M, Valente T, Bolea I, Solé M, Sun P, Benítez S, Morelló JR, Reguant J, Ramírez B, Hidalgo J, Unzeta M. Catecholaminergic and cholinergic systems of mouse brain are modulated by LMN diet, rich in theobromine, polyphenols and polyunsaturated fatty acids. Food Funct. 2015 Apr;6(4):1251-60.

152. Fernandez-Martinez MN, Hernandez-Echevarria L, Sierra-Vega M, Diez-Liebana MJ, Calle-Pardo A, Carriedo-Ule D, Sahagún-Prieto AM, Anguera-Vila A, Garcia-Vieitez JJ. A randomised clinical trial to evaluate the effects of Plantago ovata husk in Parkinson patients: changes in levodopa pharmacokinetics and biochemical parameters. BMC Complement Altern Med. 2014 Aug 12;14:296.

153. Ferry P, Johnson M, Wallis P. Use of complementary therapies and non-prescribed medication in patients with Parkinson's disease. Postgrad Med J 2002; 78:612-614

154. Fertl E, Doppelbauer A, Auff E. Physical activity and sports in patients suffering from Parkinson's disease in comparison with healthy seniors. J Neural Transm Park Dis Dement Sect 1993;5(2):157-61.

155. Field T. Violence and touch deprivation in adolescents. Adolescence 2002; 37:735-49.

156. Field T, Ironson G, Scafjdi F, Nawrocki T, Goncalves A, Burman I, Pickens J, Fox N, Schanberg S, Kuhn C. Massage therapy reduces anxiety and enhances EEG pattern of alertness and math computations. Int J Neurosci 1996; 86:197-205.

157. Flint Beal M, Henshaw DR, Jenkins BG, Rosen BR, Schulz JB. Coenzyme Q10 and nicotinamide block striatal lesions produced by the mitochondrial toxin malonate. Ann Neurol. 1994;36:882-888.

158. Flint Beal M, Matthews RT. Coenzyme Q10 in the central nervous system and its potential usefulness in the treatment of neurodegenerative diseases. Mol Aspects Med. 1997;18(S);s169-s179.

159. Flint Beal M, Matthews RT, Tieleman A, Shults CW. Coenzyme Q10 attenuates the 1-methyl-4-phenyl-1,2,3,6-tetrahydropyridine (MPTP) induced loss of striatal dopamine and dopaminergic axons in aged mice. Brain Res. 1998;783:109-114

160. Food and Drug Administration (FDA. Complementary and Alternative Medicine Products and their Regulation by the Food and Drug Administration». Office of Policy and Planning, Office of the Commissioner, Dept. of Health and Human Services, US Government. 2007. Plantilla:PD-notice

161. Formisano,R., Pratesi, L., Modarelli, F., Bonefati, V., Meco, G. (1992). Rehabilitation and parkinson's disease. Scandinavian Journal of Rehabilitation and Medicine, 24; 157-160.

162. Frazier LD. Coping with disease-related stressors in Parkinson's disease. Gerontologist. 2000 Feb;40(1):53-63.

163. Frecska E1, Bokor P2, Winkelman M3. The Therapeutic Potentials of Ayahuasca: Possible Effects against Various Diseases of Civilization. Front Pharmacol. 2016 Mar 2;7:35.

164. Fungeld EW. A natural and broad spectrum nootropic substance for treatment of SDAT—the Ginkgo biloba extract. Prog Clin Biol Res 1989;317:1247-60.

165. Fusco S, Pani G. Brain response to calorie restriction. Cell Mol Life Sci. 2013;70:3157-70.

166. Fusco S, Ripoli C, Podda MV, Ranieri SC, Leone L, Toietta G, McBurney MW, Schütz G, Riccio A, Grassi C, Galeotti T, Pani G. A role for neuronal cAMP responsive-element binding (CREB)-1 in brain responses to caloric restriction. Proc Natl Acad Sci U S A. 2012 Jan 10;109(2):621-6.

167. Gale CR, Braidwood EA, Winter PD, Martyn CN. Mortality from Parkinson's disease and other causes in men who were prisoners of war in the Far East. Lancet. 1999 Dec 18-25;354(9196):2116-8.

168. Galluzzi S, Zanetti O, Binetti G, Trabucchi M, Frisoni GB. Coma in a patient with Alzheimer's disease taking low dose trazodone and gingko biloba. J Neurol Neurosurg Psychiatry. 2000 May;68(5):679-80.

169. Gao J, Wang WY, Mao YW, Gräff J, Guan JS, Pan L, Mak G, Kim D, Su SC, Tsai LH. A novel pathway regulates memory and plasticity via SIRT1 and miR-134. Nature 2010;466:1105-9.

170. Garcia JJ, Fernandez N, Carriedo D, Diez MJ, Sahagun A, Gonzalez A, Calle A, Sierra M. Hydrosoluble fiber (Plantago ovata husk) and levodopa I: experimental study of the pharmacokinetic interaction. Eur Neuropsychopharmacol. 2005 Oct;15(5):497-503.

171. Gardner CD, Zehnder JL, Rigby AJ, Nicholus JR, Farquhar JW. Effect of Ginkgo biloba (EGb 761) and aspirin on platelet aggregation and platelet function analysis among older adults at risk of cardiovascular disease: a randomized clinical trial. Blood Coagul Fibrinolysis. 2007 Dec;18(8):787-93.

172. Gerdeman G, Lovinger DM. CB1 cannabinoid receptor inhibits synaptic release of glutamate in rat dorsolateral striatum. J Neurophysiol. 2001 Jan;85(1):468-71.

173. Gómez del Rio MA, Sánchez-Reus MI, Iglesias I, Pozo MA, García-Arencibia M, Fernández-Ruiz J, García-García L, Delgado M, Benedí J. Neuroprotective Properties of Standardized Extracts of Hypericum perforatum on Rotenone Model ofParkinson's Disease. CNS Neurol Disord Drug Targets. 2013 Aug;12(5):665-79.

174. González-Burgos E, Fernandez-Moriano C, Gómez-Serranillos MP. Potential neuroprotective activity of Ginseng in Parkinson's disease: a review. J Neuroimmune Pharmacol. 2015 Mar;10(1):14-29.

175. González-Maldonado R. El extraño caso del Dr. Parkinson. Grupo Editorial Universitario, Granada 1997.

176. González-Maldonado R. Mucuna contra Parkinson,tratamiento con levodopa natural. North Charleston: CreateSpace; 2014.

177. González-Maldonado R. Parkinson y estrés. North Charleston: CreateSpace; 2013.

178. González-Maldonado R. Tratamientos heterodoxos en la enfermedad de Parkinson. North Charleston: CreateSpace; 2013.

179. González-Maldonado R, González-Redondo R, Di Caudo C. Beneficio de la combinación de mucuna, té verde y levodopa/benseracida en la enfermedad de Parkinson. Rev Neurol 2016; 62:525-526.

180. González-Maldonado R, González-Redondo R, Di Caudo C. The clinical effects of mucuna and green tea in combination with levodopa-benserazide in advanced Parkinson's disease: Experience from a case report. International Parkinson and Movement Disorders Society, Berlin june 2016. Mov Disord 2016; 31 Suppl 2, pp. S639.

181. Gorkow C, Wuttke W, Marz RW. [Effectiveness of Vitex agnus-castus preparations]. Wien Med Wochenschr 2002;152(15-16):364-72

182. Goutopoulos A, Makriyannis A. From cannabis to cannabinergics: new therapeutic opportunities. Pharmacol Ther 2002 Aug;95(2):103-17.

183. Grantham C, Geerts H. The rationale behind cholinergic drug treatment for dementia related to cerebrovascular disease. J Neurol Sci. 2002 Nov 15;203-204:131-6.

184. Greene SM, Griffin WA. Symptom study in context: effects of marital quality on signs of Parkinson's disease during patient-spouse interaction. Psychiatry. 1998 Spring;61(1):35-45.

185. Griffin WA, Greene SM. Social interaction and symptom sequences: a case study of orofacial bradykinesia exacerbation in Parkinson's disease during negative marital interaction. Psychiatry. 1994 Aug;57(3):269-74.

186. Grunblatt E, Mandel S, Maor G, et al. Gene Expression Analysis in N-methyl-4-phenyl-1,2,3,6-tetrahydropyridine Mice Model of Parkinson's Disease Using cDNA Microarray: Effect of R-Apomorphine. J Neurochem. 2001;78:1-12.

187. Grundmann O, Wähling C, Staiger C, Butterweck V. Anxiolytic effects of a passion flower (Passiflora incarnata L.) extract in the elevated plus maze in mice. Pharmazie. 2009 Jan;64(1):63-4.

188. Grundmann O, Wang J, McGregor GP, Butterweck V. Anxiolytic activity of a phytochemically characterized Passiflora incarnata extract is mediated via the GABAergic system. Planta Med. 2008 Dec;74(15):1769-73. doi: 10.1055/s-0028-1088322. Epub 2008 Nov 12.

189. Guerranti R, Aguiyi JC, Errico E, Pagani R, Marinello E. Effects of Mucuna pruriens extract on activation of prothrombin by Echis carinatus venom. J Ethnopharmacol 2001;75:175-180.

190. Guggenheim M. Dioxypheniylalanin, eine neue Aminosäure aus Vicia faba. Z Physiol Chem 1913; 88:276-284.

191. Guo S, Yan J, Yang T, Yang X, Bezard E, Zhao B. Protective effects of green tea polyphenols in the 6-OHDA rat model of Parkinson's disease through inhibition of ROS-NO pathway. Biol Psychiatry. 2007 Dec 15;62(12):1353-62. Epub 2007 Jul 12.

192. Hadfield N. The role of aromatherapy massage in reducing anxiety in patients with malignant brain tumours. Int J Palliat Nurs. 2001 Jun;7(6):279-85.

193. Haglin L, Selander B. [Diet in Parkinson disease]. Tidsskr Nor Laegeforen. 2000;120(5):576-8.

194. Haltenhof H, Krakow K, Zofel P, Ulm G, Buhler KE. [Coping behaviors in Parkinson's disease]. Nervenarzt. 2000 Apr;71(4):275-81.

195. Hammond DC, Kabbani S. Neurohypnosis. En: Weintraub MI (ed.)Alternative and complementary treatment in neurologic illness. Churchill Livingstone, New York 2001.

196. Haneishi E. Effects of a music therapy voice protocol on speech intelligibility, vocal acoustic measures, and mood of individuals with Parkinson's disease. J Music Ther. 2001 Winter;38(4):273-90.

197. Harkey MR, Henderson GL, Gershwin ME, Stern JS, Hackman RM. Variability in commercial ginseng products: an analysis of 25 preparations. Am J Clin Nutr 2001

198. Hashiguchi M, Ohta Y, Shimizu M, Maruyama J, Mochizuki M. Meta-analysis of the efficacy and safety of Ginkgo biloba extract for the treatment of dementia. J Pharm Health Care Sci 2015;1:14.

199. Head RJ, McLennan PL, Raederstorff D, Muggli R, Burnard SL, McMurchie EJ. Prevention of nerve conduction deficit in diabetic rats by polyunsaturated fatty acids. Am J Clin Nutr 2000; 71(1Suppl):386S-392S.

200. Helland IB, Smith L, Saarem K, Saugstad OD, Drevon CA. Maternal supplementation with very-long-chain n-3 fatty acids during pregnancy and lactation augments children's IQ at 4 years of age. Pediatrics. 2003 Jan;111(1):e39-44

201. Hellenbrand W, Seidler A, Boeing H, Robra BP, Vieregge P, Nischan P, Joerg J, Oertel WH, Schneider E, Ulm G. Diet and Parkinson's disease. I: A possible role for the past intake of specific foods and food groups. Results from a self-administered food-frequency questionnaire in a case-control study. Neurology 1996 Sep;47(3):636-43. (b)

202. Henderson L, Yue QY, Bergquist C, Gerden B, Arlett P. St John's wort (Hypericum perforatum): drug interactions and clinical outcomes. Br J Clin Pharmacol 2002 Oct;54(4):349-56.

203. Heo JH, Lee ST, Chu K, Oh MJ, Park HJ, Shim JY, Kim M. Heat-processed ginseng enhances the cognitive function in patients with moderately severe Alzheimer's disease. Nutr Neurosci. 2012 Nov;15(6):278-82.

204. Hermann W. Significance of hyperhomocysteinemia. Clin Lab. 2006;52(7-8):367-74.

205. Herrschaft H, Nacu A, Likhachev S, Sholomov I, Hoerr R, Schlaefke S. Ginkgo biloba extract EGb 761® in dementia with neuropsychiatric features: a randomised, placebo-controlled trial to confirm the efficacy and safety of a daily dose of 240 mg. J Psychiatr Res. 2012 Jun;46(6):716-23.

206. Hilbert JE, Sforzo GA, Swensen T. The effects of massage on delayed onset muscle soreness. Br J Sports Med. 2003 Feb;37(1):72-5.

207. Hindmarch I, Quinlan PT, Moore KL, Parkin C. The effects of black tea and other beverages on aspects of cognition and psychomotor performance. Psycho-pharmacology (Berl). 1998;139:230-8.

208. Hirsch MA, Iyer SS, Sanjak M. Exercise-induced neuroplasticity in human Parkinson's disease: What is the evidence telling us? Parkinsonism Relat Disord. 2016 Jan;22 Suppl 1:S78-81.

209. Hobert I. Libro completo de Medicina natural. Gaia Ediciones, Madrid 1999.

210. Holland B, Pokorny ME. Slow stroke back massage: its effect on patients in a rehabilitation setting. Rehabil Nurs. 2001 Sep-Oct;26(5):182-6.

211. Homberg V. Motor training in the therapy of Parkinson's disease. Neurology 1993; 43:S45-6.

212. Homola S. Skeptical Inquirer 2003; 1.

213. Hornykiewicz O. L-DOPA: From a biologically inactive amino acid to a successful therapeutic agent Historical review article. Amino Acids 2002;23(1-3):65-70.

214. Hosamani R, Krishna G, Muralidhara. Standardized Bacopa monnieri extract ameliorates acute paraquat-induced oxidative stress, and neurotoxicity in prepubertal mice brain. Nutr Neurosci. 2014 Aug 25. [Epub ahead of print].

215. Hosamani R, Muralidhara. Neuroprotective efficacy of Bacopa monnieri against rotenone induced oxidative stress and neurotoxicity in Drosophila melanogaster. Neurotoxicology 2009;30:977-85.

216. Howarth AL. Will aromatherapy be a useful treatment strategy for people with multiple sclerosis who experience pain? Complement Ther Nurs Midwifery. 2002 Aug;8(3):138-41.

217. Howe GW. Neurological trauma and family functioning: toward a social neuropsychology. Psychiatry. 1994 Aug;57(3):275-7.

218. Howitz KT, Bitterman KJ, Cohen HY, Lamming DW, Lavu S, Wood JG, Zipkin RE, Chung P, Kisielewski A,Zhang LL, Scherer B, Sinclair DA. Small molecule activators of sirtuins extend Saccharomyces cerevisiae lifespan. Nature. 2003 Sep 11;425(6954):191-6.

219. Hu XW, Qin SM, Li D, Hu LF, Liu CF. Elevated homocysteine levels in levodopa-treated idiopathic Parkinson's disease: a meta-analysis. Acta Neurol Scand. 2013 Aug;128(2):73-82.

220. Huber K, Superti-Furga G. After the grape rush: sirtuins as epigenetic drug targets in neurodegenerative disorders. Bioorg Med Chem. 2011 Jun 15;19(12):3616-24.

221. Hurwitz A. The benefit of a home exercise regimen for ambulatory Parkinson's disease patients. J Neurosci Nurs 1989 Jun;21(3):180-4.

222. Hussain G, Manyam, BV. Mucuna pruriens proves more effective than L-DOPA in Parkinson's disease animal model. Phytotherapy Research 1997;11:419-23.

223. Ihl R, Bachinskaya N, Korczyn AD, Vakhapova V, Tribanek M, Hoerr R, Napryeyenko O; GOTADAY Study Group. Efficacy and safety of a once-daily formulation of Ginkgo biloba extract EGb 761 in dementia with neuropsychiatric features: a randomized controlled trial. Int J Geriatr Psychiatry. 2011 Nov;26(11):1186-94.

224. Ihl R, Tribanek M, Bachinskaya N; GOTADAY Study Group. Efficacy and tolerability of a once daily formulation of Ginkgo biloba extract EGb 761® in Alzheimer's disease and vascular dementia: results from a randomised controlled trial. Pharmacopsychiatry. 2012 Mar;45(2):41-6.

225. Ishige K, Schubert D, Sagara Y. Flavonoids protect neuronal cells from oxidative stress by three distinct mechanisms. Free Radic Biol Med 2001 Feb 15;30(4):433-46.

226. Ishikawa T, Funahashi T, Kudo J. Effectiveness of the Kampo kami-shoyo-san (TJ-24) for tremor of antipsychotic-induced parkinsonism. Psychiatry Clin Neurosci 2000;54:579-582.

227. Izzo AA, Ernst E. Interactions between herbal medicines and prescribed drugs: a systematic review. Drugs 2001;61:2163-2175.

228. Jadiya P, Khan A, Sammi SR, Kaur S, Mir SS, Nazir A. Anti-Parkinsonian effects of Bacopa monnieri: insights from transgenic and pharmacological Caenorhabditis elegans models of Parkinson's disease. Biochem Biophys Res Commun. 2011 Oct 7;413(4):605-10.

229. Jagatha B, Mythri RB, Vali S, Bharath MM. Curcumin treatment alleviates the effects of glutathione depletion in vitro and in vivo: therapeutic implications for Parkinson's disease explained via in silico studies. Free Radic Biol Med. 2008 Mar 1;44(5):907-17.

230. Jansen RL, Brogan B, Whitworth AJ, Okello EJ. Effects of five Ayurvedic herbs on locomotor behaviour in a Drosophila melanogaster Parkinson's disease model. Phytother Res. 2014 Dec;28(12):1789-95.

231. Jarry H, Leonhardt S, Gorkow C, Wuttke W. In vitro prolactin but not LH and FSH release is inhibited by compounds in extracts of Agnus castus: direct evidence for a dopaminergic principle by the dopamine receptor assay. Exp Clin Endocrinol 1994;102:448-454

232. Jarvis MJ. Does caffeine intake enhance absolute levels of cognitive performance? Psychopharmacology (Berl). 1993; 110:45-52.

233. Jayaraj RL, Elangovan N, Manigandan K, Singh S, Shukla S. CNB-001 a novel curcumin derivative, guards dopamine neurons in MPTP model of Parkinson's disease. Biomed Res Int. 2014;2014:236182.

234. Jawna-Zboinska K, Blecharz-Klin K, Joniec-Maciejak I, Wawer A, Pyrzanowska J, Piechal A, Mirowska-Guzel D, Widy-Tyszkiewicz E. Passiflora incarnata L. improves spatial memory, reduces stress, and affects neurotransmission in rats. Phytother Res. 2016 Jan 27.

235. Jellin JM, Gregory P, Batz F, Hitchens K, et al. Natural Medicines Comprehensive Database. Therapeutic Research. Stockton, CA. Green Tea et Black Tea. www.naturaldatabase.com

236. Jellinger KA. Cell death mechanisms in neurodegeneration. J Cell Mol Med 2001; 5:1-17.

237. Jeong KH, Jeon MT, Kim HD, Jung UJ, Jang MC, Chu JW, Yang SJ, Choi IY, Choi MS, Kim SR. Nobiletin protects dopaminergic neurons in the 1-methyl-4-phenylpyridinium-treated rat model of Parkinson's disease. J Med Food. 2015 Apr;18(4):409-14.

238. Ji HF, Shen L. The multiple pharmaceutical potential of curcumin in Parkinson's disease. CNS Neurol Disord Drug Targets. 2014 Mar;13(2):369-73.

239. Jiang TF, Zhang YJ, Zhou HY, Wang HM, Tian LP, Liu J, Ding JQ, Chen SD. Curcumin ameliorates the neurodegenerative pathology in A53T ?-synuclein cell model of Parkinson's disease through the downregulation of mTOR/p70S6K signaling and the recovery of macroautophagy. J Neuroimmune Pharmacol. 2013 Mar;8(1):356-69.

240. Jiang L, Su L, Cui H, Ren J, Li C. [Ginkgo biloba extract for dementia: a systematic review]. Shanghai Arch Psychiatry. 2013 Feb;25(1):10-21.

241. Jiang W, Wang Z, Jiang Y, Lu M, Li X. Ginsenoside Rg1 Ameliorates Motor Function in an Animal Model of Parkinson's Disease. Pharmacology. 2015;96(1-2):25-31.

242. Jimenez-Jimenez FJ, Mateo D, Gimenez-Roldan S. Premorbid smoking, alcohol consumption, and coffee drinking habits in Parkinson's disease: a case-control study. Mov Disord 1992 Oct;7(4):339-44.

243. Jin F, Wu Q, Lu YF, Gong QH, Shi JS. Neuroprotective effect of resveratrol on 6-OHDA-induced Parkinson's disease in rats. Eur J Pharmacol. 2008 Dec 14;600(1-3):78-82.

244. Johnson CC, Gorell JM, Rybicki BA, Sanders K, Peterson EL. Adult nutrient intake as a risk factor for Parkinson's disease. Int J Epidemiol 1999 Dec;28(6):1102-9.

245. Joshi J, Ghaisas S, Vaidya A, Vaidya R, Kamat DV, Bhagwat AN, Bhide S. Early human safety study of turmeric oil (Curcuma longa oil) administered orally in healthy volunteers. J Assoc Physicians India. 2003 Nov;51:1055-60.

246. Joy CB, Mumby-Croft R, Joy LA. Polyunsaturated fatty acid (fish or evening primrose oil) for schizophrenia. Cochrane Database Syst Rev. 2000;(2):CD001257.

247. Judelson DA, Preston AG, Miller DL, Muñoz CX, Kellogg MD, Lieberman HR. Effects of theobromine and caffeine on mood and vigilance. J Clin Psychopharmacol 2013 33:499-506.

248. Jun YL, Bae CH, Kim D, Koo S, Kim S. Korean Red Ginseng protects dopaminergic neurons by suppressing the cleavage of p35 to p25 in a Parkinson's disease mouse model. J Ginseng Res 2015; 39:148-54.

249. Jung UJ, Kim SR. Effects of naringin, a flavanone glycoside in grapefruits and citrus fruits, on the nigrostriatal dopaminergic projection in the adult brain. Neural Regen Res 2014;9:1514-7.

250. Junghanns K, Veltrup C, Wetterling T. Craving shift in chronic alcoholics. Eur Addict Res 2000; 6:64-70.

251. Jurado-Coronel JC, Ávila-Rodriguez M, Echeverria V, Hidalgo OA, Gonzalez J, Aliev G, Barreto GE1. Implication of Green Tea as a Possible Therapeutic Approach for Parkinson Disease. CNS Neurol Disord Drug Targets. 2016;15(3):292-300.

252. Kaada B. [Nocebo--the opposite of placebo]. Tidsskr Nor Laegeforen. 1989;109:814-21.

253. Kamel F, Goldman SM, Umbach DM, Chen H, Richardson G, Barber MR, Meng C, Marras C, Korell M, Kasten M, Hoppin JA, Comyns K, Chade A, Blair A, Bhudhikanok GS, Webster Ross G0, William Langston J, Sandler DP, Tanner CM. Dietary fat intake, pesticide use, and Parkinson's disease. Parkinsonism Relat Disord. 2014 Jan;20(1):82-7.

254. Kang KS, Wen Y, Yamabe N, Fukui M, Bishop SC, Zhu BT. Dual beneficial effects of (-)-epigallocatechin-3-gallate on levodopa methylation and hippocampal neurodegeneration: in vitro and in vivo studies. PLoS One. 2010 Aug 5;5(8):e11951.

255. Kang KS, Yamabe N, Wen Y, Fukui M, Zhu BT. Beneficial effects of natural phenolics on levodopa methylation and oxidative neurodegeneration. Brain Res. 2013 Feb 25;1497:1-14.

256. Kanowski S, Hoerr R. Ginkgo biloba extract EGb 761 in dementia: intent-to-treat analyses of a 24-week, multi-center, double-blind, placebo-controlled, randomized trial. Pharmacopsychiatry. 2003 Nov;36(6):297-303.

257. Kasdan ML, Lewis K, Bruner A, Johnson AL. The nocebo effect: do no harm. J South Orthop Assoc. 1999 Summer;8(2):108-13.

258. Kathuria S, Gaetani S, Fegley D, Valino F, Duranti A, Tontini A, Mor M, Tarzia G, Rana GL, Calignano A, Giustino A, Tattoli M, Palmery M, Cuomo V, Piomelli D. Modulation of anxiety through blockade of anandamide hydrolysis. Nat Med 2002 Dec 2; [epub ahead of print]

259. Katzenschlager R, Evans A, Manson A, Patsalos PN, Ratnaraj N, Watt H, Timmermann L, Van der Giessen R, Lees AJ. Mucuna pruriens in Parkinson's disease: a double blind clinical and pharmacological study. J Neurol Neurosurg Psychiatry. 2004 Dec;75(12):1672-7.

260. Kellogg J. The art of massage. TEACH Services, Brushton, NY 1999.

261. Kempster PA, Bogetic Z, Secombei JW, Martin HD, Balazs NDH, Wahlqvist ML (1993). Motor effects of broad beans (Vicia faba) in Parkinson's disease: single dose studies. Journal of Asia Pacific Clinical Nutrition, 2, 85-89.

262. Kempster PA, Wahlqvist ML. Dietary factors in the management of Parkinson's disease. Nutr Rev 1994;52:51–8.

263. Kennedy DO, Scholey AB, Wesnes KA. Modulation of cognition and mood following administration of single doses of Ginkgo biloba, ginseng, and a ginkgo/ginseng combination to healthy young adults. Physiol Behav 2002; 75:739-751.

264. Kikuchi A, Yamagughi H, Tanida M, Abe T. Effects of odors on cardiac response patterns and subjective states in a reaction time task.Tohoku Psychologica Folia, Vol 51, 1992, 74-82.

265. Kim CS, Park JB, Kim KJ, Chang SJ, Ryoo SW, Jeon BH. Effect of Korea red ginseng on cerebral blood flow and superoxide production. Acta Pharmacol Sin 2002;23:1152-6.

266. Kim HD, Jeong KH, Jung UJ, Kim SR. Naringin treatment induces neuroprotective effects in a mouse model of Parkinson's disease in vivo, but not enough to restore the lesioned dopaminergic system. J Nutr Biochem. 2016 Feb;28:140-6.

267. Kim HG, Ju MS, Shim JS, Kim MC, Lee SH, Huh Y, Kim SY, Oh MS. Mulberry fruit protects dopaminergic neurons in toxin-induced Parkinson's disease models. Br J Nutr 2010;104:8-16.

268. Kim MH, Kim SH, Yang WM. Mechanisms of action of phytochemicals from medicinal herbs in the treatment of Alzheimer's disease. Planta Med. 2014 Oct;80(15):1249-58.

269. Kim MS, Lee JI, Lee WY, Kim SE. Neuroprotective effect of Ginkgo biloba L. extract in a rat model of Parkinson's disease. Phytother Res. 2004; 18(8): 663–6.

270. Kim S, Ahn K, Oh TH, Nah SY, Rhim H. Inhibitory effect of ginsenosides on NMDA receptor-mediated signals in rat hippocampal neurons. Biochem Biophys Res Commun 2002; 296:247-54.

271. Kim YK, Guo Q, Packer L. Free radical scavenging activity of red ginseng aqueous extracts. Toxicology 2002 Mar 20;172(2):149-56.

272. Klemm WR, Lutes SD, Hendrix DV, Warrenburg S. Topographical EEG maps of human response to odors. Chemical Senses 1992; 17: 347-361.

273. Kloszewska I. [Acetylcholinesterase inhibitors--beyond Alzheimer's disease]. Psychiatr Pol 2002; 36 (6 Suppl):133-141.

274. Kneafsey R. The therapeutic use of music in a care of the elderly setting: a literature review. J Clin Nurs. 1997 Sep;6(5):341-6.

275. Koepp MJ, Gunn RN, Lawrence AD, Cunningham VJ, Dagher A, Jones T, Brooks DJ, Bench CJ, Grasby PM. Evidence for striatal dopamine release during a video game. Nature 1998;393:266-8.

276. Kostic VS, Svetel M, Sternic N, Dragasevic N, Przedborski S. Theophylline increases "on" time in advanced parkinsonian patients. Neurology 1999 Jun 10;52(9):1916

277. Koutrouby R. Massage Therapy: The Power of Structured Touch. Healthlogy 2002 (april 16); Editorial Review.

278. Krenn L. [Passion Flower (Passiflora incarnata L.) -a reliable herbal sedative]. Wien Med Wochenschr 2002;152(15-16):404-6.

279. Kulkarni SK, Akula KK, Deshpande J. Evaluation of antidepressant-like activity of novel water-soluble curcumin formulations and St. John's wort in behavioral paradigms of despair. Pharmacology. 2012;89(1-2):83-90.

280. Kuroda K, Tatara K, Takatorage T. Effect of Physical exercise on mortality in patients with parkinson's disease. Acta Neurol Scand 1992; 86:55-59.

281. Lakhan SE, Vieira KF. Nutritional and herbal supplements for anxiety and anxiety-related disorders: systematic review. Nutr J. 2010 Oct 7;9:42.

282. Langsjoen PH, Langsjoen AM. Overview of the use of CoQ10 in cardiovascular disease. Biofactors. 1999;9(2-4):273-84.

283. Langsjoen P, Langsjoen A, Willis R, and Folkers K. The Aging Heart: Reversal of Diastolic Dysfunction Through the Use of Oral CoQ10 in the Elderly. En: Klatz RM and Goldman R (eds.). Anti-Aging Medical Therapeutics. Health Quest Publications. 1997;113-120.

284. Lao CD, Ruffin MT 4th, Normolle D, Heath DD, Murray SI, Bailey JM, Boggs ME, Crowell J, Rock CL, Brenner DE. Dose escalation of a curcuminoid formulation. BMC Complement Altern Med 2006;6:10.

285. Lau YS, Patki G, Das-Panja K, Le WD, Ahmad SO. Neuroprotective effects and mechanisms of exercise in a chronic mouse model of Parkinson's disease with moderate neurodegeneration. Eur J Neurosci. 2011 Apr;33(7):1264-74.

286. Leanderson J; Eriksson E; Nilsson C; Wykman A. Proprioception in classical ballet dancers. A prospective study of the influence of an ankle sprain on proprioception in the ankle joint. Am J Sports Med. 1996 May-Jun. 24(3). P 370-4.

287. Le Bars PL, Katz MM, Berman N, Itil TM, Freedman AM, Schatzberg AF. A placebo-controlled, double-blind, randomized trial of an extract of Ginkgo biloba for dementia. North American EGb Study Group. JAMA. 1997 Oct 22-29;278(16):1327-32.

288. Le Bars PL, Kieser M, Itil KZ. A 26-week analysis of a double-blind, placebo-controlled trial of the ginkgo biloba extract EGb 761 in dementia. Dement Geriatr Cogn Disord. 2000 Jul-Aug;11(4):230-7.

289. Le Bars PL, Velasco FM, Ferguson JM, Dessain EC, Kieser M, Hoerr R. Influence of the severity of cognitive impairment on the effect of the Gnkgo biloba extract EGb 761 in Alzheimer's disease. Neuropsychobiology. 2002;45(1):19-26.

290. Levine BL. Singing and Parkinson's disease. Wpda. APDA Newsletter Winter 1996.

291. Liotti M, Ramig LO, Vogel D, New P, Cook Cl, Ingham RJ, Ingham JC, Fox PT. Hypophonia in Parkinson's disease: neural correlates of voice treatment revealed by PET. Neurology. 2003; 60:432-440.

292. Izzo AA, Ernst E. Interactions between herbal medicines and prescribed drugs: a systematic review. Drugs 2001;61:2163-2175.

293. Le Couteur DG, Solon-Biet S, Cogger VC, Mitchell SJ, Senior A, de Cabo R, Raubenheimer D, Simpson SJ. The impact of low-protein high-carbohydrate diets on aging and lifespan. Cell Mol Life Sci. 2016 Mar;73(6):1237-52.

294. Lecrubier Y, Clerc G, Didi R, Kieser M. Efficacy of St. John's wort extract WS 5570 in major depression: a double-blind, placebo-controlled trial. Am J Psychiatry 2002 Aug;159(8):1361-6.

295. Lee JH, Kim SR, Bae CS, Kim D, Hong H, Nah S. Protective effect of ginsenosides, active ingredients of Panax ginseng, on kainic acid-induced neurotoxicity in rat hippocampus. Neurosci Lett 2002; 325:129-133

296. Lee KS, Lee BS, Semnani S, Avanesian A, Um CY, Jeon HJ, Seong KM, Yu K, Min KJ, Jafari M. Curcumin extends life span, improves health span, and modulates the expression of age-associated aging genes in Drosophila melanogaster. Rejuvenation Res. 2010 Oct;13(5):561-70.

297. Lee WH, Loo CY, Bebawy M, Luk F, Mason RS, Rohanizadeh R. Curcumin and its derivatives: their application in neuropharmacology and neuroscience in the 21st century. Curr Neuropharmacol. 2013 Jul;11(4):338-78.

298. Leem E, Nam JH, Jeon MT, Shin WH, Won SY, Park SJ, Choi MS, Jin BK, Jung UJ, Kim SR. Naringin protects the nigrostriatal dopaminergic projection through induction of GDNF in a neurotoxin model of Parkinson's disease. J Nutr Biochem. 2014 Jul;25(7):801-6.

299. Lees A, Olanow WC, Der Giessen RV, Wagner H.Mucuna pruriens and extracts thereof for the treatment of neurological diseases. Patent WO 2004039385-A2, 2004, May 13.

300. Levites Y, Amit T, Mandel S, Youdim MB. Neuroprotection and neurorescue against Abeta toxicity and PKC-dependent release of nonamyloidogenic soluble precursor protein by green tea polyphenol (-)-epigallocatechin-3-gallate. FASEB J. 2003; 17:952-954.

301. Levites Y, Amit T, Youdim MB, Mandel S. Involvement of protein kinase C activation and cell survival/ cell cycle genes in green tea polyphenol (-)-epigallocatechin 3-gallate neuroprotective action. J Biol Chem 2002 Aug 23;277(34):30574-80 (a)

302. Levites Y, Youdim MB, Maor G, Mandel S. Attenuation of 6-hydroxydopamine (6-OHDA)-induced nuclear factor-kappaB (NF-kappaB) activation and cell death by tea extracts in neuronal cultures. Biochem Pharmacol 2002 Jan 1;63(1):21-9 (b)

303. Levites Y, Weinreb O, Maor G, Youdim MB, Mandel S. Green tea polyphenol(-)-epigallocatechin-3-gallate prevents N-methyl-4-phenyl-1,2,3,6-tetrahydropyridine-induced dopaminergic neuro-degeneration. J Neurochem 2001 Sep;78(5):1073-1082.

304. Lieberman A. Coenzyme Q10 and neuroprotection. NPF, 2002. Adaptación de: Lansjoen PH. Introduction to coenzyme Q10.

305. Lieberman HR. The effects of ginseng, ephedrine, and caffeine on cognitive performance, mood and energy. Nutr Rev 2001; 59:91-102. Review.

306. Lieu CA, Kunselman AR, Manyam BV, Venkiteswaran K, Subramanian T. A water extract of Mucuna pruriens provides long-term amelioration of parkinsonism with reduced risk for dyskinesias. Parkinsonism Relat Disord. 2010 Aug;16(7):458-65.

307. Lieu CA, Venkiteswaran K, Gilmour TP, Rao AN, Petticoffer AC, Gilbert EV, Deogaonkar M, Manyam BV, Subramanian T. The Antiparkinsonian and Antidyskinetic Mechanisms of Mucuna pruriens in the MPTP-Treated Nonhuman Primate. Evid Based Complement Alternat Med. 2012;2012:840247.

308. Lim I, van Wegen E, de Goede C, Deutekom M, Nieuwboer A, Willems A, Jones D, Rochester L, Kwakkel G. Effects of external rhythmical cueing on gait in patients with Parkinson's disease: a systematic review. Clin Rehabil. 2005 Oct;19(7):695-713.

309. Liu X, Liu F, Yue R, Li Y, Zhang J, Wang S, Zhang S, Wang R, Shan L, Zhang W. The antidepressant-like effect of bacopaside I: possible involvement of the oxidative stress system and the noradrenergic system. Pharmacol Biochem Behav. 2013 Sep;110:224-30.

310. Liu J, Wang LN, Zhan SY, Xia Y. WITHDRAWN: Coenzyme Q10 for Parkinson's disease. Cochrane Database Syst Rev. 2012 May 16;5:CD008150.

311. Logroscino G, Marder K, Cote L, Tang MX, Shea S, Mayeux R. Dietary lipids and antioxidants in Parkinson's disease: a population-based, case-control study. Ann Neurol 1996 Jan;39(1):89-94.

312. Logroscino G, Marder K, Graziano J, Freyer G, Slavkovich V, Lojacono N, Cote L, Mayeux R. Dietary iron, animal fats, and risk of Parkinson's disease. Mov Disord 1998;13 Suppl 1:13-6.

313. Lokk J. The effects of mountain exercise in Parkinsonian persons - a preliminary study. Arch Gerontol Geriatr. 2000 Aug 1;31(1):19-25.

314. Long J, Gao H, Sun L, Liu J, Zhao-Wilson X. Grape extract protects mitochondria from oxidative damage and improves locomotor dysfunction and extends lifespan in a Drosophila Parkinson's disease model. Rejuvenation Res. 2009 Oct;12(5):321-31.

315. Lötzke D,, Ostermann T,, Büssing A,. Argentine tango in Parkinson disease -a systematic review and meta-analysis. BMC Neurol. 2015 Nov 5;15:226. doi: 10.1186/s12883-015-0484-0.

316. Ludvigson H, Rottman T. Effects of ambient odors of lavender and cloves on cognition, memory, affect and mood. Chemical Sense 1989; 14: 525-536.

317. Luo FC, Wang SD, Qi L, Song JY, Lv T, Bai J. Protective effect of panaxatriol saponins extracted from Panax notoginseng against MPTP-induced neurotoxicity in vivo. J Ethnopharmacol 2011;133:448-53.

318. Luquin MR. Modelos experimentales de enfermedad de Parkinson. Rev Neurol 2000; 31:60-66.

319. Lyon MR, Cline JC, Totosy de Zepetnek J, Shan JJ, Pang P, Benishin C. Effect of the herbal extract combination Panax quinquefolium and Ginkgo biloba on attention-deficit hyperactivity disorder: a pilot study. J Psychiatry Neurosci 2001 May;26(3):221-8.

320. Macdiarmid JI, Hetherington MM. Mood modulation by food: an exploration of affect and cravings in 'chocolate addicts'. Br J Clin Psychol. 1995 Feb;34 (Pt 1):129-38.

321. Macht M, Ellgring H. Behavioral analysis of the freezing phenomenon in Parkinson's disease: a case study. J Behav Ther Exp Psychiatry. 1999 Sep;30(3):241-7.

322. Maher NE, Golbe LI et al. The GenePD Study. Epidemiologic Study of 203 sibling pairs with Parkinson's disease. Neurology 2002; 58:79-84.

323. Mak JC. Potential role of green tea catechins in various disease therapies: progress and promise. Clin Exp Pharmacol Physiol. 2012 Mar;39(3):265-73.

324. Mandel SA, Amit T, Kalfon L, Reznichenko L, Youdim MB. Targeting multiple neurodegenerative diseases etiologies with multimodal-acting greentea catechins. J Nutr. 2008 Aug;138(8):1578S-1583S.

325. Mandel SA, Amit T, Weinreb O, Reznichenko L, Youdim MB. Simultaneous manipulation of multiple brain targets by green tea catechins: a potential neuroprotective strategy for Alzheimer and Parkinson diseases. CNS Neurosci Ther. 2008 Winter;14(4):352-65.

326. Mandel SA, Amit T, Weinreb O, Youdim MB. Understanding the broad-spectrum neuroprotective action profile of green teapolyphenols in aging and neurodegenerative diseases. J Alzheimers Dis. 2011;25(2):187-208.

327. Mally J. [Most frequent causes for hand tremor in clinical practice]. Orv Hetil 1995; 136:2211-2216.

328. Mally J, Stone TW. The effect of theophylline on parkinsonian symptoms. J Pharm Pharmacol 1994; 46:515-517.

329. Mansouri Z1, Sabetkasaei M, Moradi F, Masoudnia F, Ataie A. Curcumin has neuroprotection effect on homocysteine rat model of Parkinson. J Mol Neurosci. 2012 Jun;47(2):234-42.

330. Manyam BV. Beans (Mucuna Pruriens) for Parkinson's disease: an herbal alternative. http://www.parkinson.org/beans.htm (2003).

331. Manyam BV. Paralysis agitans and levodopa in "Ayurveda": ancient Indian medical treatise. Mov Disord 1990;5:47-8

332. Manyam BV, Dhanasekaran M, Hare TA.Effect of antiparkinson drug HP-200 (Mucuna pruriens) on the central monoaminergic neurotransmitters. Phytother Res 2004; 18:97-101.

333. Manyam BV, Sanchez-Ramos JR. Traditional and complementary therapies in Parkinson's disease. Adv Neurol 1999; 80:565-574.

334. Marrelli M, Statti G, Conforti F, Menichini F. New Potential Pharmaceutical Applications of Hypericum Species. Mini Rev Med Chem 2016;16(9):710-20.

335. Markowitz JS, DeVane CL. The emerging recognition of herb-drug interactions with a focus on St. John's wort (Hypericum perforatum). Psychopharmacol Bull 2001 Winter;35(1):53-64.

336. Marsicano G, Goodenough S, Monory K, Hermann H, Eder M, Cannich A, Azad SC, Cascio MG, Gutierrez SO, van der Stelt M, Lopez-Rodriguez ML, Casanova E, Schutz G, Zieglgansberger W, Di Marzo V, Behl C, Lutz B. CB1 cannabinoid receptors and on-demand defense against excitotoxicity. Science 2003; 302:84-88.

337. Martin A, Youdim K, Szprengiel A, Shukitt-Hale B, Joseph J. Roles of vitamins E and C on neurodegenerative diseases and cognitive performance. Nutr Rev 2002 Oct;60(10 Pt 1):308-26.

338. Martín-Fernández JJ, Carles-Díes R, Cañizares F, Parra S, Avilés F, Villegas I, Morsi-Hassan O, Fernández-Barreiro A, Herrero MT. Homocisteína y deterioro cognitivo en la enfermedad de Parkinson. Rev Neurol. 2010 Feb 1-15;50(3):145-51.

339. Marwick Ch. Music that charms for care of premies. JAMA 2000; 283:468-468.

340. Marwick Ch. Music therapist in with data on medical results. JAMA 2000; 283:731-733.

341. Matthews Rt, Yang L, Browne S, Baik M, Flint Beal M. Coenzyme Q10 administration increases brain mitochondrial concentrations and exerts neuroprotective effects. Proc Natl Acad Sci 1998;95: 8892-8897.

342. Mathur D, Goyal K, Koul V, Anand A. The Molecular Links of Re-Emerging Therapy: A Review of Evidence of Brahmi (Bacopamonniera). Front Pharmacol. 2016 Mar 4;7:44..

343. Matson N. Made of stone: a view of Parkinson 'off' periods. Psychol Psychother 2002;75:93-9.

344. Mattson MP. Dietary factors, hormesis and health. Ageing Res Rev 2008;7:43-8.

345. Mattson MP. Gene-diet interactions in brain aging and neurodegenerative disorders. Ann Intern Med. 2003 Sep 2;139(5 Pt 2):441-4.

346. Mattson MP. Neuroprotective signaling and the aging brain: take away my food and let me run. Brain Res 2000 Dec 15;886(1-2):47-53.

347. Mattson MP. Will caloric restriction and folate protect against AD and PD? Neurology 2003; 60:690-695 (b)

348. Mattson MP, Chan SL, Duan W. Modification of brain aging and neurodegenerative disorders by genes, diet, and behavior. Physiol Rev 2002; 82:637-72.

349. Mattson MP, Duan W, Chan SL, Cheng A, Haughey N, Gary DS, Guo Z, Lee J, Furukawa K. Neuroprotective and neurorestorative signal transduction mechanisms in brain aging: modification by genes, diet and behavior. Neurobiol Aging 2002 Sep-Oct;23(5):695.

350. Mattson MP, Kruman II, Duan W. Folic acid and homocysteine in age-related disease. Ageing Res Rev 2002 Feb;1(1):95-111.

351. Mattson MP, Shea TB. Folate and homocysteine metabolism in neural plasticity and neurodegenerative disorders. Trends Neurosci. 2003 Mar;26(3):137-46.

352. Maurer K, Ihl R, Dierks T, Frölich L. Clinical efficacy of Ginkgo biloba special extract EGb 761 in dementia of the Alzheimer type. J Psychiatr Res. 1997 Nov-Dec;31(6):645-55.

353. Mavandadi S, Dobkin R, Mamikonyan E, Sayers S, Ten Have T, Weintraub D. Benefit finding and relationship quality in Parkinson's disease: a pilot dyadic analysis of husbands and wives. J Fam Psychol. 2014 Oct;28(5):728-34.

354. Mazza M, Capuano A, Bria P, Mazza S. Ginkgo biloba and donepezil: a comparison in the treatment of Alzheimer's dementia in a randomized placebo-controlled double-blind study. Eur J Neurol. 2006 Sep;13(9):981-5.

355. Mazzio E, Deiab S, Park K, Soliman KF. High throughput screening to identify natural human monoamine oxidase B inhibitors. Phytother Res. 2013 Jun;27(6):818-28.

356. McCarty MF. Does a vegan diet reduce risk for Parkinson's disease? Med Hypotheses 2001 Sep;57(3):318-23.

357. McEwen BJ. The influence of herbal medicine on platelet function and coagulation: a narrative review. Semin Thromb Hemost. 2015 Apr;41(3):300-14.

358. Meaney MJ, Aitken DH, Bhatnagar S, Sapolsky RM. Postnatal handling attenuates certain neuroendocrine, anatomical, and cognitive dysfunctions associated with aging in female rats. Neurobiol Aging. 1991 Jan-Feb;12(1):31-8.

359. Meaney MJ, Aitken DH, van Berkel C, Bhatnagar S, Sapolsky RM. Effect of neonatal handling on age-related impairments associated with the hippocampus. Science. 1988; 239:766-768.

360. Mechoulam R. Discovery of endocannabinoids and some random thoughts on their possible roles in neuroprotection and aggression. Prostaglandins Leukot Essent Fatty Acids 2002 Feb-Mar;66(2-3):93-9

361. Mechoulam R. Recent advantages in cannabinoid research. Forsch Komplementarmed 1999 Oct;6 Suppl 3:16-20.

362. Mechoulam R, Parker LA, Gallily R. Cannabidiol: an overview of some pharmacological aspects. J Clin Pharmacol 2002 Nov;42(11 Suppl):11S-19S.

363. Mehran S M M, Golshani B. Simultaneous determination of levodopa and carbidopa from from fava bean, green peas and green beans by high performance liquid gas chromatography. J Clin Diagn Res. 2013 Jun;7(6):1004-7.

364. Meier B, Berger D, Hoberg E, Sticher O, Schaffner W. Pharmacological activities of Vitex agnus-castus extracts in vitro. Phytomedicine 2000 Oct;7(5):373-81.

365. Melzig MF, Putscher I, Henklein P, Haber H. In vitro pharmacological activity of the tetrahydroisoquinoline salsolinol present in products from Theobroma cacao L. like cocoa and chocolate. J Ethnopharmacol 2000 Nov;73(1-2):153-9.

366. Merz PG, Gorkow C, Schrodter A, Rietbrock S, Sieder C, Loew D, Dericks-Tan JS, Taubert HD. The effects of a special Agnus castus extract (BP1095E1) on prolactin secretion in healthy male subjects. Exp Clin Endocrinol Diabetes 1996;104(6):447-53.

367. Michener W, Rozin P. Pharmacological versus sensory factors in the satiation of chocolate craving. Physiol Behav. 1994 Sep;56(3):419-22.

368. Michener W, Rozin P, Freeman E, Gale L. The role of low progesterone and tension as triggers of perimenstrual chocolate and sweets craving: some negative experimental evidence. Physiol Behav. 1999 Sep;67(3):417-20.

369. Miller GE, Cohen S, Ritchey AK. Chronic psychological stress and the regulation of pro-inflammatory cytokines: a glucocorticoid-resistance model. Health Psychol. 2002 Nov;21(6):531-41.

370. Miller JW, Selhub J, Nadeau MR, Thomas CA, Feldman RG, Wolf PA. Effect of L-dopa on plasma homocysteine in PD patients: relationship to B-vitamin status. Neurology. 2003 Apr 8;60(7):1125-9.

371. Ming JL, Kuo BI, Lin JG, Lin LC. The efficacy of acupressure to prevent nausea and vomiting in post-operative patients. J Adv Nurs. 2002 Aug;39(4):343-51.

372. Mischley LK, Allen J, Bradley R. Coenzyme Q10 deficiency in patients with Parkinson's disease. J Neurol Sci. 2012 Jul 15;318(1-2):72-5.

373. Mitchell D. Promoting enjoyment and self-belief through work rehabilitation. Arch Psychiatr Nurs. 1998 Dec;12(6):344-50.

374. Mitchell SJ, Martin-Montalvo A, Mercken EM, Palacios HH, Ward TM, Abulwerdi G, Minor RK, Vlasuk GP, Ellis JL, Sinclair DA, Dawson J, Allison DB, Zhang Y, Becker KG, Bernier M, de Cabo R. The SIRT1 activator SRT1720 extends lifespan and improves health of mice fed a standard diet. Cell Rep. 2014 Mar 13;6(5):836-43.

375. Mizumaki Y, Kurimoto M, Hirashima Y, Nishijima M, Kamiyama H, Nagai S, Takaku A, Sugihara K, Shimizu M, Endo S. Lipophilic fraction of Panax ginseng induces neuronal differentiation of PC12 cells and promotes neuronal survival of rat cortical neurons by protein kinase C dependent manner. Brain Res 2002 Sep 20;950(1-2):254-60.

376. Molina JA, Sainz-Artiga MJ, Fraile A, Jimenez-Jimenez FJ, Villanueva C, Orti-Pareja M, Bermejo F. Pathologic gambling in Parkinson's disease: a behavioral manifestation of pharmacologic treatment? Mov Disord. 2000 Sep;15(5):869-72.

377. Moller SE. Serotonin, carbohydrates and atypical depression. Pharmacol Toxicol 1992; 71 Suppl 1:61-71.

378. Montes P, Ruiz-Sanchez E, Rojas C, Rojas P1. Ginkgo biloba Extract 761: A Review of Basic Studies and Potential Clinical Use in Psychiatric Disorders. CNS Neurol Disord Drug Targets. 2015;14(1):132-49.

379. Montioli R, Voltattorni CB, Bertoldi M1. Parkinson's Disease: Recent Updates in the Identification of Human Dopa Decarboxylase Inhibitors. Curr Drug Metab. 2016;17(5):513-8.

380. Moreira A, Diógenes MJ, de Mendonça A,, Lunet N,, Barros H,. Chocolate Consumption is Associated with a Lower Risk of Cognitive Decline. J Alzheimers Dis. 2016 May 6. [Epub ahead of print]

381. Moreno Alegre V. Comunicación personal,1996.

382. Morgan A, Stevens J. Does Bacopa monnieri improve memory performance in older persons? Results of a randomized, placebo-controlled, double-blind trial. J Altern Complement Med 2010;16:753-9.

383. Morris N. The effects of lavender (Lavendula angustifolium) baths on psychological well-being: two exploratory randomised control trials. Complement Ther Med. 2002 Dec;10(4):223-8.

384. Movafegh A1, Alizadeh R, Hajimohamadi F, Esfehani F, Nejatfar M. Preoperative oral Passiflora incarnata reduces anxiety in ambulatory surgery patients: a double-blind, placebo-controlled study. Anesth Analg. 2008 Jun;106(6):1728-32.

385. Muller T. Non-dopaminergic drug treatment of Parkinson's disease. Expert Opin Pharmacother. 2001 Apr;2(4):557-72.

386. Müller T. Role of homocysteine in the treatment of Parkinson's disease. Expert Rev Neurother. 2008 Jun;8(6):957-67.

387. Muller-Vahl KR, Kolbe H, Schneider U, Emrich HM. Cannabis in movement disorders. Forsch Komplementarmed 1999 Oct;6 Suppl 3:23-7

388. Mullins P. Aromatherapy massage: its use in a ward setting. Nurs Times. 2002; 98:36-37.

389. Murphy JE, Stewart RB. Efficacy of antiparkinson agents in preventing antipsychotic-induced extrapyramidal symptoms. Am J Hosp Pharm. 1979 May;36(5):641-4.

390. Murphy LL, Lee TJ. Ginseng, sex behavior, and nitric oxide. Ann N Y Acad Sci 2002;962:372-7.

391. Myskja A, Lindbaek M. [Examples of the use of music in clinical medicine]. Tidsskr Nor Laegeforen 2000; 120:1186-1190.

392. Mythri RB, Bharath MM. Curcumin: a potential neuroprotective agent in Parkinson's disease. Curr Pharm Des. 2012;18(1):91-9.

393. Mythri RB, Veena J, Harish G, Shankaranarayana Rao BS, Srinivas Bharath MM. Chronic dietary supplementation with turmeric protects against 1-methyl-4-phenyl-1,2,3,6-tetrahydropyridine-mediated neurotoxicity in vivo: implications for Parkinson's disease. Br J Nutr. 2011 Jul;106(1):63-72.

394. Nagashayana N, Sankarankutty P, Nampoothiri MR, Mohan PK, Mohanakumar KP. Association of L-DOPA with recovery following Ayurveda medication in Parkinson's disease. J Neurol Sci 2000; 176:124-127.

395. Naliboff BD, Tachiki KH. Autonomic and skeletal muscle responses to nonelectrical cutaneous stimulation. Percept Mot Skills 1991; 72:575-584.

396. Nam SM, Choi JH, Yoo DY, Kim W, Jung HY, Kim JW, Yoo M, Lee S, Kim CJ, Yoon YS, Hwang IK. Effects of curcumin (Curcuma longa) on learning and spatial memory as well as cell proliferation and neuroblast differentiation in adult and aged mice by upregulating brain-derived neurotrophic factor and CREB signaling. J Med Food. 2014 Jun;17(6):641-9.

397. Napryeyenko O1, Borzenko I; GINDEM-NP Study Group. Ginkgo biloba special extract in dementia with neuropsychiatric features. A randomised, placebo-controlled, double-blind clinical trial. Arzneimittelforschung. 2007;57(1):4-11.

398. Napryeyenko O, Sonnik G, Tartakovsky I. Efficacy and tolerability of Ginkgo biloba extract EGb 761 by type of dementia: analyses of a randomised controlled trial. J Neurol Sci 2009;283:224-9.

399. Nassiri-Asl M, Shariati-Rad S, Zamansoltani F. Anticonvulsant effects of aerial parts of Passiflora incarnata extract in mice: involvement of benzodiazepine and opioid receptors. BMC Complement Altern Med. 2007 Aug 8;7:26.

400. National Center for Complementary and Integrative Health (NCCIH): Complementary, Alternative, or Integrative Health: what's in a name? https://nccih.nih.gov/health/integrative-health#cvsa (consultado 22/07/16)

401. Ngan A, Conduit R. A double-blind, placebo-controlled investigation of the effects of Passiflora incarnata (passionflower) herbal tea on subjective sleep quality. Phytother Res. 2011 Aug;25(8):1153-9.

402. Nie G, Cao Y, Zhao B. Protective effects of green tea polyphenols and their major component, (-)-epigallocatechin-3-gallate (EGCG), on 6-hydroxydopamine-induced apoptosis in PC12 cells. Redox Rep 2002;7(3):171-7

403. Nocerino E, Amato M, Izzo AA. Cannabis and cannabinoid receptors. Fitoterapia 2000 Aug;71 Suppl 1:S6-S12.

404. O'Keefe JH, Vogel R, Lavie CJ, Cordain L. Exercise like a hunter-gatherer: a prescription for organic physical fitness. Prog Cardiovasc Dis. 2011 May-Jun;53(6):471-9.

405. Onaivi ES, Leonard CM, Ishiguro H, Zhang PW, Lin Z, Akinshola BE, Uhl GR. Endocannabinoids and cannabinoid receptor genetics. Prog Neurobiol 2002 Apr;66(5):307-44.

406. Ong WY1, Farooqui T2, Koh HL3, Farooqui AA2, Ling EA4. Protective effects of ginseng on neurological disorders. Front Aging Neurosci. 2015 Jul 16;7:129.

407. Ottley C. Food and mood. Nurs Stand. 2000 Sep 27-Oct 3;15(2):46-52; quiz 54-5.

408. Ouchi Y, Yoshikawa E, Futatsubashi M, Okada H, Torizuka T, Sakamoto M. Effect of simple motor performance on regional dopamine release in the striatum in Parkinson disease patients and healthy subjects: a positron emission tomography study. J Cereb Blood Flow Metab. 2002 Jun;22(6):746-52.

409. Owen AM. The effects of eating chocolate on the human brain. MRC Cognition and Brain Sciences Unit and Wolfson Brain Imaging Centre, University of Cambridge, U.K. Commissioned by Cadbury Dairy Milk, June 2002. http://www.realchocolate-realfeelings.co.uk/

410. Pacchetti C, Aglieri R, Mancini F, Martignoni E, Nappi G. Active music therapy and Parkinson's disease: methods. Funct Neurol 1998 Jan-Mar;13(1):57-67.

411. Pacchetti C, Mancini F, Aglieri R, Fundaro C, Martignoni E, Nappi G. Active music therapy in Parkinson's disease: an integrative method for motor and emotional rehabilitation. Psychosom Med 2000 May-Jun;62(3):386-393.

412. Paillard T, Rolland Y, de Souto Barreto P. Protective Effects of Physical Exercise in Alzheimer's Disease and Parkinson's Disease: A Narrative Review. J Clin Neurol. 2015 Jul;11(3):212-9.

413. Pallàs M, Casadesús G, Smith MA, Coto-Montes A, Pelegri C, Vilaplana J, Camins A. Resveratrol and neurodegenerative diseases: activation of SIRT1 as the potential pathway towards neuroprotection. Curr Neurovasc Res. 2009 Feb;6(1):70-81.

414. Palmer SL, Khanolkar AD, Makriyannis A. Natural and synthetic endocannabinoids and their structure-activity relationships. Curr Pharm Des 2000; 6:1381-1397.

415. Pan T, Fei J, Zhou X, Jankovic J, Le W. Effects of green tea polyphenols on dopamine uptake and on MPP+ -induced dopamine neuron injury. Life Sci 2003; 72:1073-1083.

416. Pan T, Jankovic J, Le W. Potential therapeutic properties of green tea polyphenols in Parkinson's disease. Drugs Aging. 2003; 20:711-721.

417. Pare S, Barr SI, Ross SE. Effect of daytime protein restriction on nutrient intakes of free-living Parkinson's disease patients. Am J Clin Nutr 1992; 55:701-707.

418. Parkinson AJ, Cruz AL, Heyward WL, Bulkow LR, Hall D, Barstaed L, Connor WE. Elevated concentrations of plasma omega-3 polyunsaturated fatty acids among Alaskan Eskimos. Am J Clin Nutr. 1994 Feb;59(2):384-8.

419. Parkinson's Disease Study Group. HP-200 in Parkinson's Disease Study Group. An alternative medicine treatment for Parkinson's disease: results of a multicenter clinical trial. J Altern Complement Med 1995; 1:249-255.

420. Parkinson Study Group QE3 Investigators, Beal MF, Oakes D, Shoulson I et al. Collaborators (208). A randomized clinical trial of high-dosage coenzyme Q10 in early Parkinson disease: no evidence of benefit. JAMA Neurol. 2014, May;71(5):543-52.

421. Pase MP, Kean J, Sarris J, Neale C, Scholey AB, Stough C. The cognitive-enhancing effects of Bacopa monnieri: a systematic review of randomized, controlled human clinical trials. J Altern Complement Med. 2012 Jul;18(7):647-52.

422. Passos PP, Borba JM, Rocha-de-Melo AP, Guedes RC, da Silva RP, Filho WT, Gouveia KM, Navarro DM, Santos GK, Borner R, Picanço-Diniz CW, Pereira A Jr, de Oliveira Costa MS, Rodrigues MC, Andrade-da-Costa BL. Dopaminergic cell populations of the rat substantia nigra are differentially affected by essential fatty acid dietary restriction over two generations. J Chem Neuroanat. 2012 Jul;44(2):66-75.

423. Pelchat ML. Food cravings in young and elderly adults. Appetite. 1997 Apr;28(2):103-13.

424. Pérez C. Paleovida. Ediciones BSA. Barcelona 2012. ISBN 9788490190975

425. Perry NS, Bollen C, Perry EK, Ballard C. Salvia for dementia therapy: review of pharmacological activity and pilot tolerability clinical trial. Pharmacol Biochem Behav. 2003 Jun;75(3):651-9.

426. Peth-Nui T1, Wattanathorn J, Muchimapura S, Tong-Un T, Piyavhatkul N, Rangseekajee P, Ingkaninan K, Vittaya-Areekul S. Effects of 12-Week Bacopa monnieri Consumption on Attention, Cognitive Processing, Working Memory, and Functions of Both Cholinergic and Monoaminergic Systems in Healthy Elderly Volunteers. Evid Based Complement Alternat Med. 2012;2012:606424.

427. Petkov VD, Mosharrof AH. Effects of standardized ginseng extract on learning, memory and physical capabilities. Am J Chin Med. 1987;15(1-2):19-29.

428. Phom L, Achumi B, Alone DP, Muralidhara, Yenisetti SC. Curcumin's neuroprotective efficacy in Drosophila model of idiopathic Parkinson's disease is phase specific: implication of its therapeutic effectiveness. Rejuvenation Res. 2014 Dec;17(6):481-9. doi: 10.1089/rej.2014.1591.

429. Phulara SC, Shukla V, Tiwari S, Pandey R. Bacopa monnieri promotes longevity in Caenorhabditis elegans under stress conditions. Pharmacogn Mag. 2015 Apr-Jun;11(42):410-6.

430. Pic-Taylor A, da Motta LG, de Morais JA, Junior WM, Santos Ade F, Campos LA, Mortari MR, von Zuben MV, Caldas ED5. Behavioural and neurotoxic effects of ayahuasca infusion (Banisteriopsiscaapi and Psychotria viridis) in female Wistar rat. Behav Processes. 2015 Sep;118:102-10.

431. Pincus JH, Barry KM. Plasma levels of amino acids correlate with motor fluctuations in parkinsonism. Arch Neurol 1987 Oct;44(10):1006-9.

432. Piomelli D, Giuffrida A, Calignano A, Rodriguez de Fonseca F. The endocannabinoid system as a target for therapeutic drugs. Trends Pharmacol Sci 2000; 21:218-224.

433. Plaitakis A, Duvoisin RC. Homer's moly identified as Galanthus nivalis L.: physiologic antidote to stra-monium poisoning. Clin Neuropharmacol 1983; 6:1-5.

434. Pluck GC, Brown RG. Apathy in Parkinson's disea-se. J Neurol Neurosurg Psychiatry 2002; 73:636-642.

435. Preece J. Introducing abdominal massage in palliative care for the relief of constipation. Complement Ther Nurs Midwifery. 2002 May;8(2):101-5

436. Proust M. Du côté de chez Swann (À la recherche du temps perdu). Salinas P (Trad.). Por el camino de Swann (En busca del tiempo perdido). Unidad Editorial. Madrid 1999.

437. Pyatigorskaya N, Gallea C, Garcia-Lorenzo D, Vidailhet M, Lehericy S. A review of the use of magnetic resonance imaging in Parkinson's disease. Ther Adv Neurol Disord. 2014 Jul;7(4):206-20.

438. Quinn C, Chandler C, Moraska A. Massage therapy and frequency of chronic tension headaches. Am J Public Health. 2002 Oct;92(10):1657-61.

439. Rai D, Bhatia G, Palit G, Pal R, Singh S, Singh HK. Adaptogenic effect of Bacopa monniera (Brahmi). Pharmacol Biochem Behav. 2003 Jul;75(4):823-30.

440. Rabey JM, Vered Y, Shabtai H, Graff E, Harsat A, Korczyn AD. Broad bean (Vicia faba) consumption and Parkinson's disease. Adv Neurol 1993;60:681-684

441. Rabey JM, Vered Y, Shabtai H, Graff E, Korczyn AD. Improvement of parkinsonian features correlate with high plasma levodopa values after broad bean (Vicia faba) consumption. J Neurol Neurosurg Psychiatry 1992; 55:725-727.

442. Rao AV, Balachandran B. Role of oxidative stress and antioxidants in neurodegenerative diseases. Nutr Neurosci 2002 Oct;5(5):291-309.

443. Raphael A. "Ahh! Aromatherapy." Delicious 1994; 12:47-48.

444. Rajabally YA, Martey J. Levodopa, vitamins, ageing and the neuropathy of Parkinson's disease. J Neurol. 2013 Nov;260(11):2844-8.

445. Rajan KE, Preethi J, Singh HK. Molecular and Functional Characterization of Bacopa monniera: A Retrospective Review. Evid Based Complement Alternat Med 2015;2015:945217.

446. Rathore P, Dohare P, Varma S, Ray A, Sharma U, Jagannathan NR, Ray M. Curcuma oil: reduces early accumulation of oxidative product and is anti-apoptogenic in transient focal ischemia in rat brain. Neurochem Res. 2008 Sep;33(9):1672-82.

447. Reay JL1, Kennedy DO, Scholey AB. Effects of Panax ginseng, consumed with and without glucose, on blood glucose levels and cognitive performance during sustained 'mentally demanding' tasks. J Psychopharmacol. 2006 Nov;20(6):771-81.

448. Remington R. Calming music and hand massage with agitated elderly. Nurs Res. 2002 Sep-Oct;51(5):317-23.

449. Renaud J1, Nabavi SF2, Daglia M3, Nabavi SM2, Martinoli MG1,4. Epigallocatechin-3-Gallate, a Promising Molecule for Parkinson's Disease? Rejuvenation Res. 2015 Jun;18(3):257-69.

450. Reutens S, Sachdev P. Homocysteine in neuropsychiatric disorders of the elderly. Int J Geriatr Psychiatry 2002 Sep;17(9):859-64.

451. Reuter I, Engelhardt M, Stecker K, Baas H. (1999). Theraputic value of exercise training in Parkinson's disease. Medicine and Science in Sports and exercise, 31, (11); 1544-1549.

452. Reuter I, Harder S, Engelhardt M, Baas H. The effect of exercise on pharmacokinetics and pharmacodynamics of levodopa. Mov Disord 2000 Sep;15(5):862-8

453. Reynolds GO, Otto MW, Ellis TD, Cronin-Golomb A. The Therapeutic Potential of Exercise to Improve Mood, Cognition, and Sleep in Parkinson's Disease. Mov Disord. 2016 Jan;31(1):23-38.

454. Riba J, Anderer P, Morte A, Urbano G, Jane F, Saletu B, Barbanoj MJ. Topographic pharmaco-EEG mapping of the effects of the South American psychoactive beverage ayahuasca in healthy volunteers. Br J Clin Pharmacol. 2002; 53:613-628.

455. Riba J, Rodriguez-Fornells A, Barbanoj MJ. Effects of ayahuasca on sensory and sensorimotor gating in humans as measured by P50 suppression and prepulse inhibition of the startle reflex, respectively. Psychopharmacology (Berl) 2002; 165:18-28.

456. Riba J, Valle M, Urbano G, Yritia M, Morte A, Barbanoj MJ. Human pharmacology of ayahuasca: subjective and cardiovascular effects, monoamine metabolite excretion, and pharmacokinetics. J Pharmacol Exp Ther. 2003 Jul;306(1):73-83.

457. Rice AS. Cannabinoids and pain. Curr Opin Investig Drugs 2001 Mar;2(3):399-414

458. Riley D, Lang AE. Practical application of a low-protein diet for Parkinson's disease. Neurology 1988; 38:1026-1031.

459. Rios Romenets S, Anang J, Fereshtehnejad SM, Pelletier A, Postuma R. Tango for treatment of motor and non-motor manifestations in Parkinson's disease: a randomized control study. Complement Ther Med. 2015 Apr;23(2):175-84.

460. Ro YJ, Ha HC, Kim CG, Yeom HA. The effects of aromatherapy on pruritus in patients undergoing hemodialysis. Dermatol Nurs. 2002 Aug;14(4):231-4, 237-8, 256; quiz 239.

461. Roberson L. The importance of touch for the patient with dementia. Home Healthc Nurse 2003; 21:16-19.

462. Roberts A, Williams J. The effect of olfactory stimulation on fluency, vividness of imagery and associated mood: A preliminary study. British J Med Psychology 1992; 65: 197-199.

463. Robinson R. Green tea offers neuroprotection in PD. Lancet 2001; 358:391.

464. Rodenburg JB, Steenbeek D, Schiereck P, Bar PR. Warm-up, stretching and massage diminish harmful effects of eccentric exercise. Int J Sports Med 1994; 15: 414-419.

465. Rodriguez-Oroz MC, Lage PM, Sanchez-Mut J, Lamet I, Pagonabarraga J, Toledo JB, García-Garcia D, Clavero P, Samaranch L, Irurzun C, Matsubara JM, Irigoien J, Bescos E, Kulisevsky J, Pérez-Tur J, Obeso JA. Homocysteine and cognitive impairment in Parkinson's disease: a biochemical, neuroimaging, and genetic study. Mov Disord. 2009 Jul 30;24(10):1437-44.

466. Rodríguez Salgado B, Gómez-Arnau Ramírez J, Sánchez Mateos D, Dolengevich Segal H. Vegetales como nuevas drogas psicoactivas: una revisión narrativa. Medwave. 2016 Jan 21;16(1):e6372.

467. Rojas P, Montes P, Rojas C, Serrano-García N, Rojas-Castañeda JC. Effect of a phytopharmaceutical medicine, Ginko biloba extract 761, in an animal model of Parkinson's disease: therapeutic perspectives. Nutrition. 2012 Nov-Dec;28(11-12):1081-8.

468. Rojas P, Serrano-García N, Mares-Sámano JJ, Medina-Campos ON, Pedraza-Chaverri J, Ogren SO. EGb761 protects against nigrostriatal dopaminergic neurotoxicity in 1-methyl-4-phenyl-1,2,3,6-tetra-hydropyridine-induced Parkinsonism in mice: role of oxidative stress. Eur J Neurosci 2008;28:41-50.

469. Roland PD, Nergård CS. [Ginkgo biloba--effect, adverse events and drug interaction].Tidsskr Nor Laegeforen. 2012 Apr 30;132(8):956-9.

470. Romero J, Garcia-Palomero E, Lin SY, Ramos JA, Makriyannis A, Fernandez-Ruiz JJ. Extrapyramidal effects of methanandamide, an analog of anandamide, the endogenous CB1 receptor ligand. Life Sci 1996; 58:1249-1257

471. Romero J, Lastres-Becker I, de Miguel R, Berrendero F, Ramos JA, Fernandez-Ruiz J. The endogenous cannabinoid system and the basal ganglia. biochemical, pharmacological, and therapeutic aspects. Pharmacol Ther 2002 Aug;95(2):137-52.

472. Rosler M. The efficacy of cholinesterase inhibitors in treating the behavioural symptoms of dementia. Int J Clin Pract Suppl. 2002 Jun;(127):20-36.

473. Rosler M, Retz W, Thome J, Riederer P. Free radicals in Alzheimer's dementia: currently available therapeutic strategies. J Neural Transm Suppl 1998;54:211-9.

474. Ross GW, Abbott RD, Petrovitch H, Morens DM, Grandinetti A, Tung KH, Tanner CM, Masaki KH, Blanchette PL, Curb JD, Popper JS, White LR. Association of coffee and caffeine intake with the risk of Parkinson disease. JAMA 2000 May 24-31;283(20):2674-9.

475. Ross GW, Petrovitch H. Current evidence for neuroprotective effects of nicotine and caffeine against Parkinson's disease. Drugs Aging 2001;18(11):797-806.

476. Routh LC, Black JL, Ahlskog JE. Parkinson's disease complicated by anxiety. Mayo Clin Proc. 1987 Aug;62(8):733-5.

477. Rozin P, Levine E, Stoess C. Chocolate craving and liking. Appetite. 1991 Dec;17(3):199-212.

478. Rozin P, Stoess C. Is there a general tendency to become addicted? Addict Behav 1993;18:81-87.

479. Rudakewich M, Ba F, Benishin CG. Neurotrophic and neuroprotective actions of ginsenosides Rb(1) and Rg(1). Planta Med 2001 Aug;67(6):533-7.

480. Russo E. Cannabis for migraine treatment: the once and future prescription? An historical and scientific review. Pain 1998 May;76(1-2):3-8

481. Sakajiri K, Takamori M. [Body fat loss in patients with Parkinson's disease]. Rinsho Shinkeigaku 1997; 37:611-4.

482. Sala F, Mulet J, Choi S, Jung SY, Nah SY, Rhim H, Valor LM, Criado M, Sala S. Effects of ginsenoside Rg2 on human neuronal nicotinic acetylcholine receptors. J Pharmacol Exp Ther 2002; 301:1052-1059.

483. Samoylenko V1, Rahman MM, Tekwani BL, Tripathi LM, Wang YH, Khan SI, Khan IA, Miller LS, Joshi VC,Muhammad I. Banisteriopsis caapi, a unique combination of MAO inhibitory and antioxidative constituents for the activities relevant to neurodegenerative disorders and Parkinson's disease. J Ethnopharmacol. 2010 Feb 3;127(2):357-67.

484. Sánchez-Ramos JR. Banisterine and Parkinson's disease. Clin Neuropharmacol 1991;14:391-402.

485. Sandroni P. Aphrodisiacs past and present: a historical review. Clin Auton Res 2001;11:303-7

486. Sanmukhani J, Satodia V, Trivedi J, Patel T, Tiwari D, Panchal B, Goel A, Tripathi CB. Efficacy and safety of curcumin in major depressive disorder: a randomized controlled trial. Phytother Res. 2014 Apr;28(4):579-85.

487. Sarris J, McIntyre E, Camfield DA. Plant-based medicines for anxiety disorders, part 2: a review of clinical studies with supporting preclinical evidence. CNS Drugs. 2013 Apr;27(4):301-19.

488. Sasaki K, Hatta S, Wada K, Ohshika H, Haga M. Bilobalide prevents reduction of gamma-aminobutyric acid levels and glutamic aciddecarboxylase activity induced by 4-O-methylpyridoxine in mouse hippocampus. Life Sci. 2000 Jun 30;67(6):709-15.

489. Scandalis TA, Bosak A, Berliner JC, Helman LL, Wells MR. Resistance training and gait function in patients with Parkinson's disease. Am J Phys Med Rehabil. 2001 Jan;80(1):38-43; quiz 44-6.

490. Scheider WL, Hershey LA, Vena JE, Holmlund T, Marshall JR, Freudenheim. Dietary antioxidants and other dietary factors in the etiology of Parkinson's disease. Mov Disord 1997 Mar;12(2):190-6

491. Schelosky L, Raffauf C, Jendroska K et al. Kava and dopamine antagonism (letter). J Neurol Neurosurg Psychiatry 1995;58:639-40.

492. Schenkman M, Cutson T, Kuchibhatla M,Chandler J, Pieper C, Ray L, Laub K. Exercise to improve spinal flexibility and function for people with parkinson's disease: a randomized, controlled trial. Journal of the American Geriatrics Society 1998; 46:1207-1216.

493. Scholey AB, Kennedy DO. Acute, dose-dependent cognitive effects of Ginkgo biloba, Panax ginseng and their combination in healthy young volunteers: differential interactions with cognitive demand. Hum Psychopharmacol 2002 Jan;17(1):35-44

494. Schroeder BE, Binzak JM, Kelley AE. A common profile of prefrontal cortical activation following exposure to nicotine- or chocolate-associated contextual cues. Neuroscience. 2001;105(3):535-45.

495. Schulz V. Clinical trials with hypericum extracts in patients with depression--results, comparisons, conclusions for therapy with antidepressant drugs. Phytomedicine 2002 Jul;9(5):468-74.

496. Schwarz MJ, Houghton PJ, Rose S, Jenner P, Lees AD. Activities of extract and constituents of Banisteriopsis caapi relevant to parkinsonism. Pharmacol Biochem Behav. 2003 Jun;75(3):627-33

497. Seet RC, Lim EC, Tan JJ, Quek AM, Chow AW, Chong WL, Ng MP, Ong CN, Halliwell B. Does high-dose coenzyme Q10 improve oxidative damage and clinical outcomes in Parkinson's disease? Antioxid Redox Signal. 2014 Jul 10;21(2):211-7.

498. Serafini M et al. Plasma antioxidants from chocolate. Nature 2003, 424:1013.

499. Sesso HD, Gaziano JM, Buring JE, Hennekens CH. Coffee and tea intake and the risk of myocardial infarction. Am J Epidemiol 1999; 149:162-167.

500. Sevcik J, Masek K. Potential role of cannabinoids in Parkinson's disease. Drugs Aging 2000; 16:391-395.

501. Shah C, Beall EB, Frankemolle AM, Penko A, Phillips MD, Lowe MJ, Alberts JL,,. Exercise Therapy for Parkinson's Disease: Pedaling Rate Is Related to Changes in Motor Connectivity. Brain Connect. 2016 Feb;6(1):25-36.

502. Shealy CN. Enciclopedia ilustrada de remedios naturales. Könemann, Köln 1999. (passim)

503. Sheikh N, Ahmad A, Siripurapu KB, Kuchibhotla VK, Singh S, Palit G. Effect of Bacopa monniera on stress induced changes in plasma corticosterone and brain monoamines in rats. J Ethnopharmacol. 2007 May 22;111(3):671-6.

504. Shen L, Liu CC, An CY, Ji HF. How does curcumin work with poor bioavailability? Clues from experimental and theoretical studies. Sci Rep. 2016 Feb 18;6:20872.

505. Shen LR1, Parnell LD, Ordovas JM, Lai CQ. Curcumin and aging. Biofactors 2013;39:133-40.

506. Shih IF, Liew Z, Krause N, Ritz B. Lifetime occupational and leisure time physical activity and risk of Parkinson's disease. Parkinsonism Relat Disord. 2016 Jul;28:112-7.

507. Shin JY, Song JY, Yun YS, Yang HO, Rhee DK, Pyo S. Immunostimulating effects of acidic polysaccharides extract of Panax ginseng on macrophage function. Immunopharmacol Immunotoxicol 2002 Aug;24(3):469-82.

508. Shinomol GK, Mythri RB, Srinivas Bharath MM, Muralidhara. Bacopa monnieri extract offsets rotenone-induced cytotoxicity in dopaminergic cells and oxidative impairments in mice brain. Cell Mol Neurobiol. 2012 Apr;32(3):455-65.

509. Sieradzan KA, Fox SH, Hill M, Dick JP, Crossman AR, Brotchie JM. Cannabinoids reduce levodopa-induced dyskinesia in Parkinson's disease: a pilot study. Neurology. 2001 Dec 11;57(11):2108-11.

510. Sikorska M, Lanthier P, Miller H, Beyers M, Sodja C, Zurakowski B, Gangaraju S, Pandey S, Sandhu JK. Nanomicellar formulation of coenzyme Q10 (Ubisol-Q10) effectively blocks ongoing neurodegeneration in the mouse 1-methyl-4-phenyl-1,2,3,6-tetrahydropyridine model: potential use as an adjuvant treatment in Parkinson's disease. Neurobiol Aging. 2014 Oct;35(10):2329-46.

511. Silverdale MA, McGuire S, McInnes A, Crossman AR, Brotchie JM. Striatal cannabinoid CB1 receptor mRNA expression is decreased in the reserpine-treated rat model of Parkinson's disease. Exp Neurol. 2001 Jun;169(2):400-6.

512. Siriwardhana N, Kalupahana NS, Moustaid-Moussa N. Health benefits of n-3 polyunsaturated fatty acids: eicosapentaenoic acid and docosahexaenoic acid. Adv Food Nutr Res. 2012;65:211-22.

513. Shobana C, Kumar RR, Sumathi T. Alcoholic extract of Bacopa monniera Linn. protects against 6-hydroxydopamine-induced changes in behavioral and biochemical aspects: a pilot study. Cell Mol Neurobiol. 2012 Oct;32(7):1099-112.

514. Shotton HR, Clarke S, Lincoln J. The effectiveness of treatments of diabetic autonomic neuropathy is not the same in autonomic nerves supplying different organs. Diabetes. 2003 Jan;52(1):157-64.

515. Shults CW, Haas RH, Passov D, Beal MF. Coenzyme Q10 levels correlate with the activities of complexes I and II/III in mitochondria from parkinsonian and nonparkinsonian subjects. Ann Neurol. 1997 Aug;42(2):261-4.

516. Shults CW, Oakes D, Kieburtz K, Beal MF, Haas R, Plumb S, Juncos JL, Nutt J, Shoulson I, Carter J, Kompoliti K, Perlmutter JS, Reich S, Stern M, Watts RL, Kurlan R, Molho E, Harrison M, Lew M; Parkinson Study Group. Effects of coenzyme Q10 in early Parkinson disease: evidence of slowing of the functional decline. Arch Neurol 2002;59:1541-50

517. Siddique YH, Jyoti S, Naz F. Effect of epicatechin gallate dietary supplementation on transgenic Drosophila model of Parkinson's disease. J Diet Suppl. 2014 Jun;11(2):121-30.

518. Siddique YH, Naz F, Jyoti S. Effect of curcumin on lifespan, activity pattern, oxidative stress, and apoptosis in the brains of transgenic Drosophila model of Parkinson's disease. Biomed Res Int. 2014;2014:606928.

519. Sinclair AJ, Murphy KJ, Li D. Marine lipids: overview "news insights and lipid composition of Lyprinol". Allerg Immunol (Paris). 2000 Sep;32(7):261-71.

520. Singh B, Singh D, Goel RK. Dual protective effect of Passiflora incarnata in epilepsy and associated post-ictal depression. J Ethnopharmacol. 2012 Jan 6;139(1):273-9.

521. Singh R, Ramakrishna R, Bhateria M, Bhatta RS. In vitro evaluation of Bacopa monniera extract and individual constituents on human recombinant monoamine oxidase enzymes. Phytother Res. 2014 Sep;28(9):1419-22.

522. Sliutz G, Speiser P, Schultz AM, Spona J, Zeillinger R. Agnus castus extracts inhibit prolactin secretion of rat pituitary cells. Horm Metab Res 1993 May;25(5):253-5.

523. Smith DG, Standing L, de Man A. Verbal memory elicited by ambient odor. Perceptual and Motor Skills 1992; 74:339-343.

524. Smith MC, Kemp J, Hemphill L, Vojir CP. Outcomes of therapeutic massage for hospitalized cancer patients. J Nurs Scholarsh. 2002;34(3):257-62.

525. Smith MC, Stallings MA, Mariner S, Burrall M. Benefits of massage therapy for hospitalized patients: a descriptive and qualitative evaluation. Altern Ther Health Med 1999; 5:64-71.

526. Smith PF, Maclennan K, Darlington CL. The neuroprotective properties of the Ginkgo biloba leaf: a review of the possible relationship to platelet-activating factor. J Ethnopharmacol. 1996; 50: 131–9.

527. Sokolova L, Hoerr R, Mishchenko T. Treatment of Vertigo: A Randomized, Double-Blind Trial Comparing Efficacy and Safety of Ginkgo biloba Extract EGb 761 and Betahistine. Int J Otolaryngol 2014; 2014:682439.

528. Solanki I, Parihar P, Mansuri ML, Parihar MS. Flavonoid-based therapies in the early management of neurodegenerative diseases. Adv Nutr. 2015 Jan 15;6(1):64-72.

529. Soler J, Elices M, Franquesa A, Barker S, Friedlander P, Feilding A, Pascual JC, Riba J. Exploring the therapeutic potential of Ayahuasca: acute intake increases mindfulness-related capacities. Psychopharmacology (Berl). 2016 Mar;233(5):823-9.

530. Song S, Nie Q, Li Z, Du G..Curcumin improves neurofunctions of 6-OHDA-induced parkinsonian rats. Pathol Res Pract. 2015 Nov 18. pii: S0344-0338(15)30042-X.

531. Song JX, Sze SC, Ng TB, Lee CK, Leung GP, Shaw PC, Tong Y, Zhang YB. Anti-Parkinsonian drug discovery from herbal medicines: what have we got from neurotoxic models? J Ethnopharmacol. 2012 Feb 15;139(3):698-711.

532. Spinelli KJ, Osterberg VR, Meshul CK, Soumyanath A, Unni VK. Curcumin Treatment Improves Motor Behavior in ?-Synuclein Transgenic Mice. PLoS One. 2015 Jun 2;10: e0128510.

533. Soulimani R, Younos C, Jarmouni S, Bousta D, Misslin R, Mortier F. Behavioural effects of Passiflora incarnata L. and its indole alkaloid and flavonoid derivatives and maltol in the mouse. J Ethnopharmacol 1997 Jun;57(1):11-20.

534. Soumyanath A, Denne T, Peterson A, Shinto L. Assessment of commercial formulations of Mucuna pruriens seeds for levodopa content. P01.36. International Research Congress on Integrative Medicine and Health, Portland, Oregon 2012. BMC Complement Altern Med 2012; 12 (Suppl 1): S36.

535. Spaulding SJ, Barber B, Colby M, Cormack B, Mick T, Jenkins ME. Cueing and gait improvement among people with Parkinson's disease: a meta-analysis. Arch Phys Med Rehabil. 2013 Mar;94(3):562-70.

536. Srivastav S, Singh SK, Yadav AK, Srikrishna S. Folic Acid Supplementation Ameliorates Oxidative Stress, Metabolic Functions and Developmental Anomalies in a Novel Fly Model of Parkinson's Disease. Neurochem Res. 2015 Jul;40(7):1350-9.

537. Srivastav S, Singh SK, Yadav AK, Srikrishna S. Folic acid supplementation rescues anomalies associated with knockdown of parkin in dopaminergic and serotonergic neurons in Drosophila model of Parkinson's disease. Biochem Biophys Res Commun. 2015 May 8;460(3):780-5.

538. Steinberg FM, Bearden MM, Keen CL. Cocoa and chocolate flavonoids: implications for cardiovascular health. J Am Diet Assoc. 2003 Feb;103(2):215-23.

539. Strathearn KE, Yousef GG, Grace MH, Roy SL, Tambe MA, Ferruzzi MG, Wu QL, Simon JE, Lila MA, Rochet JC. Neuroprotective effects of anthocyanin- and proanthocyanidin-rich extracts in cellular models of Parkinson?s disease. Brain Res. 2014 Mar 25;1555:60-77.

540. Stuckenschneider T, Helmich I, Raabe-Oetker A, Froböse I, Feodoroff B. Active assistive forced exercise provides long-term improvement to gait velocity and stride length in patients bilaterally affected by Parkinson's disease. Gait Posture. 2015 Oct;42(4):485-90.

541. Suganuma H, Hirano T, Arimoto Y, Inakuma T. Effect of tomato intake on striatal monoamine level in a mouse model of experimental Parkinson's disease. J Nutr Sci Vitaminol (Tokyo) 2002;48:251-4.

542. Sugimoto N, Miwa S, Hitomi Y, Nakamura H, Tsuchiya H, Yachie A. Theobromine, the primary methylxanthine found in Theobroma cacao, prevents malignant glioblastoma proliferation by negatively regulating phosphodiesterase-4, extracellular signal-regulated kinase, Akt/mammalian target of rapamycin kinase, and nuclear factor-kappa B. Nutr Cancer. 2014;66(3):419-23.

543. Suoh S, Donoyama N, Ohkoshi N. Anma massage (Japanese massage) therapy for patients with Parkinson's disease in geriatric health services facilities: Effectiveness on limited range of motion of the shoulder joint. J Bodyw Mov Ther. 2016 Apr;20(2):364-72.

544. Suzuki J, Yamauchi Y, Horikawa M, Yamagata S. Fasting therapy for psychosomatic diseases with special reference to its indication and therapeutic mechanism. Tohoku J Exp Med 1976;118 Suppl:245-259.

545. Talom RT, Judd SA, McIntosh DD, McNeill JR. High flaxseed (linseed) diet restores endothelial function in the mesenteric arterial bed of spontaneously hypertensive rats. Life Sci 1999;64:1415-25.

546. Tan MS, Yu JT, Tan CC, Wang HF, Meng XF, Wang C, Jiang T, Zhu XC, Tan L. Efficacy and adverse effects of ginkgo biloba for cognitive impairment and dementia: a systematic review and meta-analysis. J Alzheimers Dis. 2015;43(2):589-603.

547. Tanaka K, Galduróz RFS, Gobbi LTB, Galduróz JCF. Ginkgo Biloba Extract in an Animal Model of Parkinson's Disease: A Systematic Review. Curr Neuropharmacol 2013;11:430–435.

548. Tanji H, Anderson KE, Gruber-Baldini AL, Fishman PS, Reich SG, Weiner WJ, Shulman LM. Mutuality of the marital relationship in Parkinson's disease. Mov Disord 2008; 23: 1843-9.

549. Tavassoly O, Kakish J, Nokhrin S, Dmitriev O, Lee JS. The use of nanopore analysis for discovering drugs which bind to ?-synuclein for treatment of Parkinson's disease. Eur J Med Chem 2014;88:42-54.

550. Taylor AG, Galper DI, Taylor P, Rice LW, Andersen W, Irvin W, Wang XQ, Harrell FE Jr. Effects of adjunctive Swedish massage and vibration therapy on short-term postoperative outcomes: a randomized, controlled trial. J Altern Complement Med. 2003 Feb;9(1):77-89.

551. Taylor D, Miaskowski C, Kohn J. A randomized clinical trial of the effectiveness of an acupressure device (relief brief) for managing symptoms of dysmenorrhea. J Altern Complement Med 2002;8(3):357-70.

552. Tellone E, Galtieri A, Russo A, Giardina B, Ficarra S. Resveratrol: A Focus on Several Neurodegenerative Diseases. Oxid Med Cell Longev. 2015;2015:392169.

553. Tessitore A, Ahariri AR, Fera F, Smith WG, Chase TN, Hyde TM, Weinberger DR, Mattay VS. Dopamine Modulates the Response of the Human Amygdala: A Study in Parkinson's Disease. J Neuroscience 2002, 22:9099-9103

554. Tessitore A, Giordano A, De Micco R, Russo A, Tedeschi G. Sensorimotor connectivity in Parkinson's disease: the role of functional neuroimaging. Front Neurol 2014;5:180.

555. Thacker EL, Chen H, Patel AV, McCullough ML, Calle EE, Thun MJ, Schwarzschild MA, Ascherio A. Recreational physical activity and risk of Parkinson's disease. Mov Disord. 2008 Jan;23(1):69-74.

556. Thaut MH, Kenyon GP, Schauer ML, McIntosh GC. The connection between rhythmicity and brain function. IEEE Eng Med Biol Mag. 1999 Mar-Apr;18(2):101-8.

557. Ticinesi A,, Meschi T,, Lauretani F, Felis G, Franchi F, Pedrolli C, Barichella M, Benati G0, Di Nuzzo S, Ceda GP,, Maggio M,. Nutrition and Inflammation in Older Individuals: Focus on Vitamin D, n-3 Polyunsaturated Fatty Acids and Whey Proteins. Nutrients. 2016 Mar 29;8(4). pii: E186.

558. Toy WA, Petzinger GM, Leyshon BJ, Akopian GK, Walsh JP, Hoffman MV, Vu?kovi? MG, Jakowec MW. Treadmill exercise reverses dendritic spine loss in direct and indirect striatal medium spiny neurons in the 1-methyl-4-phenyl-1,2,3,6-tetrahydropyridine (MPTP) mouse model of Parkinson's disease. Neurobiol Dis. 2014 Mar;63:201-9.

559. Triantafyllou NI, Kararizou E, Angelopoulos E, Tsounis S, Boufidou F, Evangelopoulos ME, Nikolaou C, Vassilopoulos D. The influence of levodopa and the COMT inhibitor on serum vitamin B12 and folate levels in Parkinson's disease patients. Eur Neurol. 2007;58(2):96-9.

560. Triantafyllou NI, Nikolaou C, Boufidou F, Angelopoulos E, Rentzos M, Kararizou E, Evangelopoulos ME, Vassilopoulos D. Folate and vitamin B12 levels in levodopa-treated Parkinson's disease patients: their relationship to clinical manifestations, mood and cognition. Parkinsonism Relat Disord. 2008;14(4):321-5.

561. Tripanichkul W1, Jaroensuppaperch EO. Ameliorating effects of curcumin on 6-OHDA-induced dopaminergic denervation, glial response, and SOD1 reduction in the striatum of hemiparkinsonian mice. Eur Rev Med Pharmacol Sci. 2013 May;17(10):1360-8.

562. Tripanichkul W, Jaroensuppaperch EO. Curcumin protects nigrostriatal dopaminergic neurons and reduces glial activation in 6-hydroxydopamine hemiparkinsonian mice model. Int J Neurosci. 2012 May;122(5):263-70.

563. Tsay SL, Chen ML. Acupressure and quality of sleep in patients with end-stage renal disease: a randomized controlled trial. Int J Nurs Stud 2003; 40:1-7. (a),

564. Tsay SL, Rong JR, Lin PF. Acupoints massage in improving the quality of sleep and quality of life in patients with end-stage renal disease. J Adv Nurs. 2003 Apr;42(2):134-42. (b)

565. Tuomisto T, Hetherington MM, Morris MF, Tuomisto MT, Turjanmaa V, Lappalainen R. Psychological and physiological characteristics of sweet food "addiction". Int J Eat Disord. 1999 Mar;25(2):169-75.

566. Tuon T, Valvassori SS, Dal Pont GC, Paganini CS, Pozzi BG, Luciano TF, Souza PS, Quevedo J, Souza CT, Pinho RA. Physical training prevents depressive symptoms and a decrease in brain-derived neurotrophic factor in Parkinson's disease. Brain Res Bull. 2014 Sep;108:106-12.

567. Tytgat J, Van Boven M, Daenens P. Cannabinoid mimics in chocolate utilized as an argument in court. Int J Legal Med 2000;113(3):137-9.

568. Vaidya AB, Rajagopalan TG, Mankodi NA, Antarkar DS, Tathed PS, Purohit AV, Wadia NH. Treatment of Parkinson's disease with the cowhage plant-Mucuna pruriens Bak. Neurol India 1978; 26:171-176

569. Valkovic P, Benetin J, Blazícek P, Valkovicová L, Gmitterová K, Kukumberg P. Reduced plasma homocysteine levels in levodopa/entacapone treated Parkinson patients. Parkinsonism Relat Disord. 2005 Jun;11(4):253-6.

570. van Dongen M, van Rossum E, Kessels A, Sielhorst H, Knipschild P. Ginkgo for elderly people with dementia and age-associated memory impairment: a randomized clinical trial. J Clin Epidemiol. 2003 Apr;56(4):367-76.

571. Van Kampen JM, Baranowski DB, Shaw CA, Kay DG. Panax ginseng is neuroprotective in a novel progressive model of Parkinson's disease. Exp Gerontol. 2014 Feb;50:95-105.

572. Van Kampen J, Robertson H, Hagg T, Drobitch R. Neuroprotective actions of the ginseng extract G115 in two rodent models of Parkinson's disease. Exp Neurol. 2003 Nov;184(1):521-9.

573. Vazquez I, Aguera-Ortiz LF. Herbal products and serious side effects: a case of ginseng-induced manic episode. Acta Psychiatr Scand 2002 Jan;105(1):76-7; discussion 77-8.

574. Veerendra Kumar MH, Gupta YK. Effect of different extracts of Centella asiatica on cognition and markers of oxidative stress in rats. J Ethnopharmacol. 2002;79(2):253-60.

575. Verdery RB, Ingram DK, Roth GS, Lane MA. Caloric restriction increases HDL2 levels in rhesus monkeys (Macaca mulatta). Am J Physiol. 1997 Oct;273(4 Pt 1):E714-9.

576. Verna R. The history and science of chocolate. Malays J Pathol. 2013 Dec;35(2):111-21.

577. Vernay D, Eschalier A, Durif F, Aumaitre O, Rigal B, Ben Sadoun A, Fialip J, Marty H, Philip E, Bougerolle AM, et al. [Salsolinol, an endogenous molecule. Possible implications in alcoholism, Parkinson's disease and pain]. Encephale 1989 Nov-Dec;15(6):511-6.

578. Vieregge P, von Maravic C, Friedrich HJ. Life-style and dietary factors early and late in Parkinson's disease. Can J Neurol Sci 1992 May;19(2):170-3.

579. Viliani T, Pasquetti P, Magnolfi S, Lunardelli ML, Giorgi C, Serra P, Taiti PG. Effects of physical training on straightening-up processes in patients with Parkinson's disease. Disabil Rehabil 1999; 21:68-73.

580. Villeponteau B, Cockrell R, Feng J. Nutraceutical interventions may delay aging and the age-related diseases. Exp Gerontol 2000 Dec;35(9-10):1405-17.

581. Vilming ST. [Diet therapy in Parkinson disease]. Tidsskr Nor Laegeforen 1995 Apr 20;115(10):1244-7.

582. Virmani A, Pinto L, Binienda Z, Ali S. Food, nutrigenomics, and neurodegeneration-neuroprotection by what you eat! Mol Neurobiol. 2013 Oct;48(2):353-62.

583. Wahl D, Cogger VC, Solon-Biet SM, Waern RV, Gokarn R, Pulpitel T, Cabo R, Mattson MP, Raubenheimer D, Simpson SJ, Le Couteur DG. Nutritional strategies to optimise cogni-tive function in the aging brain. Ageing Res Rev. 2016. pii: S1568-1637(16)30054-X.

584. Wang JY, Yang JY, Wang F, Fu SY, Hou Y, Jiang B, Ma J, Song C, Wu CF. Neuroprotective effect of pseudoginsenoside-f11 on a rat model of Parkinson's disease induced by 6-hydroxydopamine. Evid Based Complement Alternat Med. 2013;2013:152798.

585. Wang Y, Xu H, Fu Q, Ma R, Xiang J. [Resveratrol derived from rhizoma et radix polygoni cuspidati and its liposomal form protect nigral cells of Parkinsonian rats]. [Article in Chinese]. Zhongguo Zhong Yao Za Zhi. 2011 Apr;36(8):1060-6. RESUMEN PUBMED

586. Wang YH, Samoylenko V, Tekwani BL, Khan IA, Miller LS, Chaurasiya ND, Rahman MM, Tripathi LM, Khan SI, Joshi VC,Wigger FT, Muhammad I. Composition, standardization and chemical profiling of Banisteriopsis caapi, a plant for the treatment of neurodegenerative disorders relevant to Parkinson's disease. J Ethnopharmacol. 2010 Apr 21;128(3):662-71.

587. Wang YQ, Wang MY, Fu XR, Peng-Yu, Gao GF, Fan YM, Duan XL, Zhao BL, Chang YZ, Shi ZH. Neuroprotective effects of ginkgetin against neuroinjury in Parkinson's disease model induced by MPTP via chelating iron. Free Radic Res. 2015;49(9):1069-80.

588. Watanabe K. [A case-control study of Parkinson's disease] Nippon Koshu Eisei Zasshi 1994;41:22-33.

589. Weinreb O, Mandel S, Youdim MB. cDNA gene expression profile homology of antioxidants and their antiapoptotic and proapoptotic activities in human neuroblastoma cells. FASEB J. 2003;17:935-7.

590. Weisburger JH. Lifestyle, health and disease prevention: the underlying mechanisms. Eur J Cancer Prev. 2002 Aug;11 Suppl 2:S1-7.

591. Wiley JL. Cannabis: discrimination of "internal bliss"? Pharmacol Biochem Behav 1999;64:257-260.

592. Willems-Giesbergen P. Lack of dopamine and inverse relation between addiction (smoking, alchool consumption)and parkinsonism. AAN 52nd Annual Meeting - San Diego (CA) April 29-May 6, 2000.

593. Willner P, Benton D, Brown E, Cheeta S, Davies G, Morgan J, Morgan M. "Depression" increases "craving" for sweet rewards in animal and human models of depression and craving. Psychopharmacology (Berl). 1998 Apr;136(3):272-83

594. Wilms H, Zecca L, Rosenstiel P, Sievers J, Deuschl G, Lucius R. Inflammation in Parkinson's diseases and other neurodegenerative diseases: cause and therapeutic implications. Curr Pharm Des 2007; 13:1925-8.

595. White HL, Scates PW, Cooper BR. Extracts of Ginkgo biloba leaves inhibit monoamine oxidase. Life Sci. 1996; 58:1315–21

596. Wiklund I Karlberg J Lund BA double-blind comparison of the effect on quality of life of a combination of vital substances including standardized Ginseng G 115 and placebo. Curr Ther Res 1994;55:32-42.

597. Wliklund IK, Mattsson LA, Lindgren R, Limoni C. Effects of a standardized ginseng extract on quality of life and physiological parameters in symptomatic post-menopausal women: a double-blind,placebo-controlled trial. Swedish Alternative Medicine Group. Int J Clin Pharmacol Res 1999; 19:89-99

598. Woelk H, Arnoldt KH, Kieser M, Hoerr R. Ginkgo biloba special extract EGb 761 in generalized anxiety disorder and adjustment disorder with anxious mood: a randomized, double-blind, placebo-controlled trial. J Psychiatr Res. 2007 Sep;41(6):472-80.

599. Wolz M, Kaminsky A, Löhle M, Koch R, Storch A, Reichmann H. Chocolate consumption is increased in Parkinson's disease. Results from a self-questionnaire study. J Neurol. 2009 Mar;256(3):488-92.

600. Wu WR, Zhu XZ. Involvement of monoamine oxidase inhibition in neuro-protective and neurorestorative effects of Ginkgo biloba extract against MPTP-induced nigrostriatal dopaminergic toxicity in C57 mice. Life Sci. 1999; 65(2): 157–64.

601. Wu Z, Smith JV, Paramasivam V, Butko P, Khan I, Cypser JR, Luo Y. Ginkgo biloba extract EGb 761 increases stress resistance and extends life span of Caenorhabditis elegans. Cell Mol Biol (Noisy-le-grand). 2002 Sep;48(6):725-31.

602. Xia X, Cheng G, Pan Y, Xia ZH, Kong LD. Behavioral, neurochemical and neuroendocrine effects of the ethanolic extract from Curcumalonga L. in the mouse forced swimming test. J Ethnopharmacol. 2007 Mar 21;110(2):356-63.

603. Xia X, Pan Y, Zhang WY, Cheng G, Kong LD. Ethanolic extracts from Curcuma longa attenuates behavioral, immune, and neuroendocrine alterations in a rat chronic mild stress model. Biol Pharm Bull. 2006 May;29(5):938-44.

604. Xu CL, Qu R, Zhang J, Li LF, Ma SP. Neuroprotective effects of madecassoside in early stage of Parkinson's disease induced by MPTP in rats. Fitoterapia. 2013 Oct;90:112-8.

605. Yabuki Y, Ohizumi Y, Yokosuka A, Mimaki Y, Fukunaga K. Nobiletin treatment improves motor and cognitive deficits seen in MPTP-inducedParkinson model mice. Neuroscience 2014;259:126-41.

606. Yang J, Song S, Li J2, Liang T3. Neuroprotective effect of curcumin on hippocampal injury in 6-OHDA-induced Parkinson's disease rat. Pathol Res Pract. 2014 Jun;210(6):357-62.

607. Yang J, Wang HP, Zhou L, Xu CF. Effect of dietary fiber on constipation: a meta analysis. World J Gastroenterol. 2012 Dec 28;18(48):7378-83.

608. Yang L, Jin X, Yan J, Jin Y, Yu W, Wu H, Xu S. Prevalence of dementia, cognitive status and associated risk factors among elderly of Zhejiang province, China in 2014. Age Ageing. 2016 May 21. pii: afw088.

609. Yang SF, Wu Q, Sun AS, Huang XN, Shi JS. Protective effect and mechanism of Ginkgo biloba leaf extracts for Parkinson disease induced by 1-methyl-4-phenyl-1,2,3,6-tetrahydropyridine. Acta Pharmacol Sin 2001; 22:1089-1093.

610. Yasui K, Kowa H, Nakaso K, Takeshima T, Nakashima K. Plasma homocysteine and MTHFR C677T genotype in levodopa-treated patients with PD. Neurology 2000 Aug 8;55(3):437-40.

611. Yoritaka A, Kawajiri S, Yamamoto Y, Nakahara T, Ando M, Hashimoto K, Nagase M, Saito Y, Hattori N. Randomized, double-blind, placebo-controlled pilot trial of reduced coenzyme Q10 for Parkinson's disease. Parkinsonism Relat Disord. 2015 Aug;21(8):911-6.

612. Youdim KA, Joseph JA. A possible emerging role of phytochemicals in improving age-related neurological dysfunctions: a multiplicity of effects. Free Radic Biol Med. 2001 Mar 15;30(6):583-94.

613. Youdim MB, Grunblatt E, Levites Y, Maor G, Mandel S. Early and late molecular events in neurodegeneration and neuroprotection in Parkinson's disease MPTP model as assessed by cDNA microarray; the role of iron. Neurotox Res. 2002 Nov-Dec;4(7-8):679-689.

614. Youdim MB, Yehuda S. The neurochemical basis of cognitive deficits induced by brain iron deficiency: involvement of dopamine-opiate system. Cell Mol Biol (Noisy-le-grand). 2000 May;46(3):491-500.

615. Yritia M, Riba J, Ortuno J, Ramirez A, Castillo A, Alfaro Y, de la Torre R, Barbanoj MJ. Determination of N,N-dimethyltryptamine and beta-carboline alkaloids in human plasma following oral administration of Ayahuasca. J Chromatogr B Analyt Technol Biomed Life Sci 2002; 779:271-281.

616. Yu S1, Zheng W, Xin N, Chi ZH, Wang NQ, Nie YX, Feng WY, Wang ZY. Curcumin prevents dopaminergic neuronal death through inhibition of the c-Jun N-terminal kinase pathway. Rejuvenation Res. 2010 Feb;13(1):55-64. doi: 10.1089/rej.2009.0908.

617. Zárate P, Díaz V. Aplicaciones de la musicoterapia en la medicina. Rev Méd Chile 2001; 129:219-233.

618. Zbarsky V, Datla KP, Parkar S, Rai DK, Aruoma OI, Dexter DT. Neuroprotective properties of the natural phenolic antioxidants curcumin and naringenin but not quercetin and fisetin in a 6-OHDA model of Parkinson's disease. Free Radic Res. 2005 Oct;39(10):1119-25.

619. Zhang F, Shi JS, Zhou H, Wilson B, Hong JS, Gao HM. Resveratrol protects dopamine neurons against lipopolysaccharide-induced neurotoxicity through its anti-inflammatory actions. Mol Pharmacol. 2010 Sep;78(3):466-77.

620. Zhang Y, Chen J, Qiu J, Li Y, Wang J, Jiao J. Intakes of fish and polyunsaturated fatty acids and mild-to-severe cognitive impairment risks: a dose-response meta-analysis of 21 cohort studies. Am J Clin Nutr. 2016 Feb;103(2):330-40.

621. Zhang ZX, Anderson DW, Mantel N, Roman GC. Motor-neuron disease in Guam: geographic and familial occurrence 1956-85. Acta Neurol Scand 1996; 94: 51-79.

622. Zheng W, Xiang YQ2, Ng CH3, Ungvari GS4, Chiu HF5, Xiang YT6. Extract of Ginkgo biloba for Tardive Dyskinesia: Meta-analysis of Randomized Controlled Trials. Pharmacopsychiatry. 2016 Mar 15.

623. Zhou H, Beevers CS, Huang S.The targets of curcumin. Curr Drug Targets 2011;12:332-47.

624. Zhou T, Zu G, Wang X, Zhang XG, Li S, Liang ZH, Zhao J. Immunomodulatory and neuroprotective effects of ginsenoside Rg1 in the MPTP(1-methyl-4-phenyl-1,2,3,6-tetrahydropyridine) -induced mouse model of Parkinson's disease. Int Immunopharmacol. 2015 Dec;29(2):334-43.

625. Zhou T, Zu G, Zhang X, Wang X, Li S, Gong X, Liang Z, Zhao J. Neuroprotective effects of ginsenoside Rg1 through the Wnt/?-catenin signaling pathway in both in vivo and in vitro models of Parkinson's disease. Neuropharmacology. 2016 Feb;101:480-9.

626. Zhu BT. On the mechanism of homocysteine pathophysiology and pathogenesis: a unifying hypothesis. Histol Histopathol 2002 Oct;17(4):1283-91.

627. Zigmond MJ, Smeyne RJ. Exercise: Is it a neuroprotective and if so, how does it work? Parkinsonism Relat Disord. 2014 Jan;20 Suppl 1:S123-7.

628. Zoccolella S, dell'Aquila C, Abruzzese G, Antonini A, Bonuccelli U, Canesi M, Cristina S, Marchese R, Pacchetti C, Zagaglia R, Logroscino G, Defazio G,Lamberti P, Livrea P. Hyperhomocysteinemia in levodopa-treated patients with Parkinson's disease dementia. Mov Disord 2009;24:1028-33.

629. Zoccolella S, Lamberti P, Armenise E, de Mari M, Lamberti SV, Mastronardi R, Fraddosio A, Iliceto G, Livrea P. Plasma homocysteine levels in Parkinson's disease: role of antiparkinsonian medications. Parkinsonism Relat Disord 2005 Mar;11:131-3.

630. Zollman, C. et al. (1999). «What is complementary medicine?». ABC of complementary medicine. BMJ 319(7211): 693-6.

631. http://www.msc.es/agemed/csmh/notas/hiperico.asp

632. http://www.naturaldatabase.com

633. http://www.parkinson.org (passim)

634. http://www.parkinson.org/sites/default/files/Estar_en_forma_cuenta.pdf (consultado 23/07/16)

635. http://www.wpda.org/articles/basic_mng/other(non_pharma)/massage.html

636.http://www.bastyr.edu/research/studies/complementary-alternative-medicine-care-parkinsons-disease -cam-care-pd

Table of contents

TABLE OF CONTENTS

FINIS